This book is dedicated to my wife. We had begun the journey together as teenagers, and, now as seniors, there is time for contemplation of what passed.

It was her support and love which made home base a place of sanity, when all else appeared, not so. Sometimes, perhaps many, I forgot to say thanks. Truth is, there is no way to say this, for all that she has done, and meant to me. She is my soul, which is truly needed at times, in my profession.

She has been my guide through life, and will never know she deserved better.

NOT UNDERSTANDING THE CHALLENGE

The concept of this book has reverberated for years, in my idle thoughts.
Now a senior, I had time to reflect upon my growth in medicine, and lives crossed.
So many "amazing stories" I have witnessed.

The journey, was not what I expected.
It certainly changed my view of others, and of the world.
I'll be the first to admit, I am a one, or zero, person. I seldom see the world in the broad spectrum of a rainbow, but rather in, a yes or no.
Even now, I see no reason to apologize for such bent, since it has served me so well. But, I must reflect, the world does not always fit into my notions.

So where to begin?
For a start, I am willing to admit my middle class background, and nurturing parents, imbibed me with a sense of entitlement. I see myself now, as the exact opposite, a convert to the harsh school of reality.
It was wonderful to grow up oblivious to the facts of life, protected and loved.
I thought of my parents as very authoritarian. Who doesn't when young?
And I was smart, which enabled me to be intellectually lazy. This did not work out so well.
My mother inspired me to adventure and the impossible. My dad, an accountant by trade, had his feet on the ground, and brought an insurance policy for any

immature behavior.

As a child, I remember wanting first to be an Archaeologist, then Astronaut (that title didn't even exist), Physicist, and then about second grade,

a NEUROSURGEON !

Why, if people asked? Because it is the hardest thing to do!

You notice right now, there was a disconnect at what I considered hard, and what I was willing to bring to the table.

This was surprisingly not realized by me, not just as a second grader, but well into my medical career. Let's just consider the term once more "naive." In retrospect, you would think terms "oblivious or stupid," as more accurate.

I'm convinced that this is not the typical path for a neurosurgeon. So don't cancel your appointment to see one, if scheduled. The other Neurosurgeons I know, have always been highly motivated to work from an early age.

It won't make my story any less amusing, however. Because although this may be a story about "my journey," the patients I encountered, are the ones that defined this. They are the real story.

Furthermore, it is not humility (which admittedly is not my strong suit) that prompts me to put pen to paper (alright laptop), but the poignancy, humor, and absurdity, and tragedy, of these encounters throughout my career. Some managed to combine all of the above.

We're in College now. Pre med.

I plan to do this in three years, rather than the typical four, for a degree.

And, this was accomplished. But even then, something seemed out of kilter.

I observed my friends to be taking this trip much more seriously than myself.

Reflecting back on those years as a B+ student, I would conclude, I neither worked hard, or played hard. Considering my minimal achievements at the time, it would have suggested far more leisure accomplishments.

I got by.

Medical school was different.

Same friends, smart boys and girls, but they were definitely in a different place than me. They were smart, I was smart, but they knew how to study, and I didn't.

A real awakening, but not enough to change my ways.

I wasn't Interested in medicine.

Here's the punch line.

I just wanted to become a neurosurgeon!

Biochemistry, just didn't seem too pertinent, likewise microbiology.

And, in my defense, the idea of grading on a curve where 25% was an A, and 15% a D (at least on one exam, I remembered) seemed absurd.

Opinion: there should be a "core" curriculum for training physicians that they must get a 100%. Repeat the testing until this is achieved.

It was a guessing game with a hundred pages a day to consume at times, and "guess" which facts "were really" worth remembering.

This wasn't going to happen.

But it was the system.

Somehow I survived. There is a God.

Third year medical student, first year with patient contact.

White short coat, check. New medical toys (stethoscope, BP cuff, ophthalmoscope, reflex hammer) check. County hospital with wards of patients, commonly 30 men on one side, 30 women on the other,…interesting. Doctors washroom (cleaned and used only by us) lab, and nursing station between.

There's a different world out there Charlie!

Reporting for duty Miss, I addressed some Nurse, not recalled.

Your instructions?

Glancing half my way, "take this chart, and exam Mr. so and so, bed 7."

Will do! Look mom, I can act like a real physician, and do an honest day's work.

Good day Sir, began my new life.

I'm a medical student, who would like to do an exam on you.

May I ask your problem Sir?

I'm going to die now.

"What"?

Say again.

We take a pause here for the reader to understand, my memories of such events, though distant, are seared into my soul. They actually happened! I couldn't forget them, should I live to be a hundred (barring Alzheimer's).

Veterans of wars probably can relate.

He stops breathing, starring at me forever.

Someone quick, get a doctor!

Code Blue, Nurses, staff, maybe an intern.

Moment later, no prolonged chest thumping, or airbag, it's all over.

I'm left standing. An observer, wondering what just happened?

Is it all going to be like this?

Chapter 2.   A Step Into the Darkness.

With respect, I would caution readers that the following pages
contain graphic descriptions of terrible illnesses and injuries.
Also, it may appear on initial observation, that there is lack of sympathy
or compassion for those in most need. I did not attempt to sugar
coat or adjust these descriptions, because they represent the accurate
memories and impressions of a shell shocked young man.
Finally, some of these events will appear so outlandish, than one could
suspect fabrication from this author. Rest assured, I observed all
described, except events specifically mentioned as possible Urban
(County hospital) legends.
It is my belief and hope, that such institutions no longer exist in our country
However, you can only judge yourself the possibilities in less developed
regions of this world.

The patients demanded pity.
This is a horror show. Look, I'm not offended, but don't tell me, I can't laugh.
Alright then, these patients are the exception, not reality. If it was the latter,
 I don't think I could wrap my mind about all of this.
A county hospital guarantees experience not seen in others!
That's why we are here. You will see things in one year, you might not see

In ten, or ever, in a typical practice.

Traveling on.

I get to stay in the hospital at night (sharing a room with a number of other lost souls) if I can find a bed at 2 AM, to be paged at 3AM, for another task. The lights are off in these on-call rooms, and beds are "as available", so careful where you touch!

Cool.

I'm important. I'm needed.

Assigned to a surgical ward, I learned practical matters.

How to do basic lab work. Urinalysis, measuring the Hematocrit, never, ever upset the elevator man. He will make you take the stairs to the 6th floor, forever. Rumors were he owned the Cadillac always parked out front, in the No Parking Zone. Truth? I don't plan on finding out.

I see physician dishonesty (actual doctors), and worse. Somethings wrong here, and it may not be all me.

Would be smart to disappear into the walls. Who am I kidding, couldn't pursue that option, too much of an (will call it) extrovert.

A "minor" example was an intern, caught red handed, not doing a thorough physical exam, who later, on his report noted both eyes WNL (within normal limits) …
in a patient with a prosthetic eye!

The resident in charge of this fool, was not amused.

Prowling the very dark wide halls at night, to observe, to learn.

Noting the "open windows" on the top floor "IN" the surgical suites (for temperature control).

Funny wall there, a collection by physicians of all things patient's shoved up their urological and gynecological access areas. Well, didn't even know you could do that. And they were framed !   (Hint, think light bulbs, toys and even a small tool chest).

You had to be there.
Not sure this is the best place to be, if you are sick.

And how can a patient commit suicide with alternate restraints on?
These incidents did make me question the path I've taken.

But there were lighter stories, in this parody of Dante's circles.

One of such levity, occurred when walking to my car one Saturday morning, after being on call (day-night-day), with another medical student.
My dad let me use an old Pontiac Catalina for school.
I parked in an "unprotected" lot, as had all medical students.
It was ventured, should a group of local citizens be seen breaking into your vehicle, walk away, slowly.

My friend was driving a NEW Pontiac. His car was next to mine.
Now whenever, we parked, we strapped the steering wheel with a heavy chain and lock, and took the "Coil wire" out of the car (never knew what that did, except it immobilized the vehicle).

I groaned in remembering an oversight.
Christ, I forgot to pull the coil wire last night!
My friend, laughed at me, "It's gone! Don't even bother looking."

Yet, there it was! I unwound the chain, about the steering wheel, twisted the ignition key, and …nothing happened !

Puzzled, I looked out the window and saw my friend gazing out across the lot. His car was gone.

They took "my coil wire" and used it to jack his car!

Now that was funny! Alright, not so much for him.

Being stranded in the parking lot at night time however, wasn't.

I remember a bitter cold night where I couldn't get a key into the lock to open my car. I tried and tried.

Looking around constantly, I remember someone, gave me matches.

Thank God. Heating the key, then inserting it, unjammed the frozen lock.

No one was around. Sure glad.

These were all great stories to tell the next day to fellow classmates.

Better yet, was the "unbelievable trauma" seen.

You may think the following cases are exceptional, I can assure you, they were not.

Being in the ER late one night, a young man with Afro hair do came in complaining of a bad headaches after being "stabbed up there."

I didn't think much of it, until I got a simple skull x ray, which showed about a 3 inch ice pick inside the center of his head…midline.

This is not the best place to be stabbed.

I called a Neurosurgical resident, whose eyes visibly widened on seeing the films.

The patient was awake, and neurologically intact.

Are you going to remove it? I asked.

He turned back at me and looked as if I asked the craziest question in the world. "Noooo…I'll admit him, monitor him neurologically, and notify a staff neurosurgeon."

Never got follow up for that one.

Be patient with me. Some of these are half stories. There's not always an ending, in real life. Unless, it is the end of life.

A pause, to present a further description of the working environment.

Careful in the tunnels, I was told, referring to the vast subterranean labyrinth interconnecting various hospital facilities. Sometimes when it's real cold out, "homeless" will find their way in there. The heat from the prehistoric boilers, and ductwork keeps them warm. "They crawl up there. And, some don't make it. Have to be cleaned out."

"Rarely threatening," however, the resident physician grinned. Another, fanciful story? Too many of these checked out. But, never had that happen to me, or anyone I knew. Possible, maybe even likely, for some desperate souls.

Back to the Vignettes.

Fun ways not to die (at least in the 1960s). Esophageal varices from alcoholism. These are very large friable veins in your swallowing pipe. Hard to control the vast outpouring of blood if you can't get good pressure on something you can't see, even if you could get a rubber tube there, as tried.

Bleeding was profuse, choking, then death. Not pretty. I wasn't there when it happened, to one patient I was following. It would have been interesting to see the device used, in the attempt to control, what was inevitable…a skill set worth having. Hope it was quick for him.

You may note so far, I was inured to the travesties of mankind, observing them as a scientist might, who wishes to improve his knowledge base. Unfortunately, my attitude then, was probably prevalent.

Whether or not the milieu was to blame, those desperate situations did evoke sometimes graveside humor. It was necessary.

Night time in the Hospital was eerie. You might see a compatriot or two from your Medical school, to eat with, for a snack, or heaven forbid, what was called dinner. Unbelievable stories to tell "of that day."

But one night about 3 AM (a favorite time for bedtime stories) I was on the ward and needed to have a bowel movement. I walked to the physicians bathroom. A place of sanctity and cleanliness. Maybe 4 by 4 feet in size. Sitting down, I saw an animal cross in front of me, it appeared half Cockroach, half Tyrannosaurus Rex. Never seen a critter that big without a license! Pulling up my scrubs, I raced to the lab, a dozen feet away, and found the most toxic substance I could use to decimate the critter. I sealed the door with tape after pouring in the contents of a large container of its contents (I believe chloroform).

The next morning rounds began as usual.
I hoped the beggar died a slow death.
Half way through the first ward, the intern excused himself momentarily.
This was upsetting, because he had the most immediate knowledge of many
patient's care.

The Chief Resident was not amused when the intern returned a half hour later, and after visiting numerous patients. He even, made short of the absurd excuse given by the intern, that he fell asleep on the commode.

That was a good time to say nothing.

CHAPTER 3.   WAR STORIES

I suppose all these are "war stories."

Finding the word human in inhumane seemed impossible.
These were desperate patients. The quality of care poor, maybe for the time, barely acceptable. I honestly don't know how Physicians could remain on staff at that facility, for years.
Some were dedicated, and honest. Some in transit. Many I believe, just numb.

I think of the good found in some, like an anesthesiologist who had a very sore arm after a whole days work. Over, and over again. There weren't ventilators at that time in this hospital. Squeezing the bag was the way for general anesthesia, thousands and thousands of times, daily. And there were other unlikely servants of the people who did their jobs, lived their lives, and got little respect, certainly no honors, for such devotion.

But we didn't get close to patients., emotionally. Which is to say, asking about their lives, small talk. There was little time, little in common, and no professional ever encouraged this verbally, or by example.
As Charity patients, they presented with a host of injuries and illnesses not generally seen in swanky suburban hospitals. They were not just sick, they were very sick, not just shot once, or stabbed once. There was even a rumored execution of females by trans vaginal gunshot, called by the hospital's name.

It was impossible to separate fact from fiction, unless you were personal witness to an event.

Things were absurd.

And patients somehow survived with the most treacherous of all injuries, such as a knife from the eye to exit the neck (seen). Don't know how that was even possible (still had usable vision).

There was little respect for life, even then, in such a community.

And physicians, who came from a different background, found themselves unfamiliar with the talk, the poverty… the patient was an extrapolation of a certain population.

I suspect that remains today.

While having later been in the Armed Services, I never saw war action, but could now understand the indifference to one's own health, let alone others.

I found no pity, when I became the item.

I was on a couch coughing. I was desperately sick, with a high temperature.

I suspect it was Pneumonia. It was curious, laying on a leather couch in the interns "dorm". Not fancy, not pretty, probably many years old. It had seen a lot. Seemed out of place, as we all were. Somehow, I managed my duties. Barely.

When that passed, things went back to the usual for me.

I didn't learn (again). This time referring to what was needed to become that person I wanted to be, not just scholastically.

Maybe great expectations, with limited achievement.

Interesting thought. I believe it likely that some rather spectacular surgeons and internists trained in such a place. Remembered.

Still think in their dreams of the very dark corridors and tunnels.

Not many now though, most are gone.

I stop and ponder the differences then, and the present.

Patients demand they be heard today.

After all, everyone is a patient sometimes!

Of course, this doesn't always occur, even now.

But then, we were raging warriors of Medicine…the "point of the spear."

Well, at times.

At other times, we were caricatures.

An extremely obese pregnant patient is about to deliver.

I'm on the Ob/Gyne call, and the resident needs help with her.

We arrive in the delivery suite, as a baby seems to fly out.

The resident makes a good catch. But there's more. Another infant about to be delivered is seen with our high tech "flashlight".

And low and behold, never suspected by anyone, a few minutes later, a third infant joins the crowd.

An Intern, also now assisting, asks holding the flashlight, if "they might be attracted to the light." We all laugh.

The intern is a good Joe, and knows I've been there when the team needed me.

He says tomorrow is Sunday and he has part ownership in a plane.

Really? A small part, but he plans on going skiing up north in the morning. If I was willing to pay for my share of the fuel, he would take me.

Wow ! This could be the start of my fear of flying.

When off the call, I hurried to my apartment, waking a still sleeping wife, to explain my plans, and her permission (she was working as an RN), I heard. "whatever you want sweetheart."

And sped off to a day of FUN.

No broken bones, Good company. A much needed reprieve from the ever unfolding medical catastrophes.

While in College, I used every summer to accumulate credits for a BS degree within 3 years, not 4. I went to more than one college to obtain these, depending on course availability.

In Medical school, I likewise looked for opportunities to gain in Medical experience.

You see I was "driven," despite my poor study habits.

After my first year, I served as an extern in a small suburban hospital doing histories and physicals, drawing blood, assisting in the OR.

Between the second and third year I was hired by a Physiatrist with several other fellow students to do "something." (Except for working on presentations for an upcoming AMA meeting, I don't know what.)

Since this was a VA project, I'm sure it had to do with maintaining research funding.

Interesting in retrospect, where some of the items this Rehabilitation physician (Physiatrist) had in development.

One was a pen for blind people, that would enable them to "read print".

It did this by creating a sound, they would hear with earphones.

An "L" would have a short burst of all frequencies, followed by a low tone.

An "F" would again have a brief all frequency sound followed by a longer

mid and high frequency sound.

And so forth.

Never caught on.

He also had a small motor attached to a belt for people with drop foot,

and/or possible weakness in a lower extremity. When the patient stepped on

a switch with the other foot, a motor pulled a specialized brace that

the elevated contralateral limb. Very cool. Never saw that either in production.

Mind you, this was the 1960s!

Finally, between my third and fourth year I had accepted, a challenge to rotate

as an "Extern" in an out of state Charity hospital. It was much smaller,

In a smaller city, and had slightly less ill patients.

This was three months of general surgery rotation doing hard time.

I would marry my sweetheart that Autumn, and painfully said goodbye one

night, driving a thousand miles to this next experience.

During that stint, I again contacted pneumonia (probably Legionaries type).

Sleeping quarters were top floor, and for 7 days, my room had night time

temperature of 100 degrees+.

Suspect that was the reason for the illness, jumping daily to what I considered

the frosty climate of an OR. (Do you have any scrubs with fur lining?)

The first month I lost thirty pounds,

There simply was not the opportunity to eat.

One supervising physician was an intern said to "volunteer" another year in that position, for the experience. Strange?

He was aggressive. Mean spirited. Scary.

Rounds included frequent reference to the New England Journal of Medicine, quoting articles delivered allegedly by airmail the night before.

Others who received their journal in snail mail, "should know this stuff."

One-upmanship.

What was the patient's serum uranium this morning?

What?

Quit stalling, if you don't know the answer, read the article!

And don't be so ignorant. Patient's can suffer because of it. (low blow).

So in the middle of one night, he determined it was in the best interest for a lady in her eighties to have what appeared to me elective surgery. Why wait until everyone's awake? We're doing it now!

She survived. And I was left to monitor her until she fully wakened.

About 4 AM in the morning, she started crying for her mother.

I held her hand until she rested. But a few minutes later she would begin this all over again. Her mental function was obviously challenged by anesthesia, if not the surgery itself.

Then a couple hours later, just about when the hospital comes alive again, a Nurse came into the Recovery room.

She was walking past our area when a "very old lady" inquired about her daughter.

You guessed it. She was over a hundred years, and the patient was happy, mom could finally visit with her.

That could have been a good 2 hours sleep.

But now the new day begins again, bracing myself.

That physician, an intern was not the only, or certainly not, most challenging Doctor, who ruled my day.

I was especially interested in any Neurosurgical experience and actively sought out a Resident Neurosurgeon from Barcelona.

Mistake.

One night a man came in with a gunshot wound to the head.

We were told it was a 357 magnum.

Eyes fixed and dilated, the Resident rushed him to the OR to debride, and decompress his brain. The OR Tech, but especially the Anesthesiologist voiced strong concern over a man they felt was DOA.

My budding Neurosurgeon was stronger willed, and we proceeded to the OR.

Here's, where it gets to be fun.

That physician was obviously not in control, of the situation.

He handed several instruments for me to hold, not pass off, for each hand.

The scrub Tech shrugged, sympathetically.

Then it happened.

Something came loose, and he said in panic, "grab this scalpel" which he had been using!. I had no way of doing that.

I asked if I could relinquish a sucker or clamp to accomplish this.

But he would have none of that.

He suddenly struck the sharp point of the scalpel into the top part of my hand, right through the glove.

That's it ! shouted the nurse (I didn't scream to the best of my recollection).

The Anesthesiologist said "you're on your own" and was about to walk out.

For some reason, I took charge.

Pulling the knife from my gloved hand, I found little bleeding, though it was deeper than a superficial wound.

There's nothing to do but complete the job. For better or worse.

"If I am staying, everyone should stay." I told them so.

They did.

The patient was dead.

My wound was not that bad. (Never received an apology from the surgeon).

But that morning I held my head a little higher.

It would take more than that to intimidate me, from what I deemed best patient care.

I learned a lot from this experience again.

Books, still of little interest to me. Real life was. And this was that.

I needed to find a "Neurosurgery for Dummies" text, if I was to really tone up.

I did learn about motorcycles.

Another night brought three ambulances to our ER.

The first two had a man in one, and some of his limbs in the other.

 (I think an arm and one leg).

The third was his girlfriend.

Total night surgery.

He passed.

The girl survived, with horrible lacerations and fractures.

Doesn't matter who's to blame. You are vulnerable on those contraptions.

That was my conclusion.

My fourth year was not as challenging emotionally or ethically.

VA hospital, and Psych rotation.

I found myself being a little bit of a rebel (harmful to yours truly, of course).

I couldn't accept many of the psychiatric principles of the day.

I remembered being told in no subtle discussion, that a passing grade might not be considered. I even remembered the event that triggered this response.

"What enables you to be the judge of Normal"? spoken to a Psychiatrist on staff, with presumably some self confidence issues.

Live and learn.

Oh wait, that was yet to come.

But, I was personally convinced much of what was diagnosed as psychiatric, was indeed, of organic basis. More of that later. (You will see, I was way ahead of my time.)

So by now, I was recognized as, not a real great student (understatement).

While that was true, I did have my moments.

The rotation at the very large VA institution was another type of "experience".

First patient I examined very closely, ophthalmoscope my eye to his, suddenly coughed violently. " Scuse me, Tuberculosis," he replied.

We had not been given any information about that patient other then he would cooperate for a general physical exam, including close eye exam.

No problem.

But the next four patients I examined, all had a condition known as Sarcoidosis. It seemed, and is, a strange mystifying disease. I was fascinated.

Grand Rounds were always a way for some senior staff to humiliate and humble other junior staff, and impress their own diagnostic acumen upon the remainder of us peons. Another way of saying they were smart, we weren't. So one such meeting centered about a gentleman with confusing symptoms. Other Junior staff were bewildered. The residents from Internal Medicine also had no clue. The Presenter was all smiles. He turned to the interns in hope of further humiliating their betters, but still no answer.
Indeed this case was fascinating.
Finally he turned to the medical students, of which I was one. He asked if any would venture an opinion. None did. These were some pretty smart guys. I had no clue.

Unfortunately, as the Lion sees the Gazelle, I caught his eye.
What do you think? He asked pointedly. My fellow students, could barely restrain themselves.
Aaaa, Sarcoidosis? I asked.
He stepped back.
How did you know?
I replied with the audiences eyes on me. "What else could it be?"
He pursued me no further accomplishing his task of destroying those that should have known.
In retrospect, maybe my reply wasn't so stupid after all.

Nope. It wasn't a turning point for me yet.

INTERLUDE

So in the 1960s, we (medical students, interns, residents) were told how easy our life was… "when I was a resident, and so forth." It will seem strange to reflect on this idea over the next few chapters.

Indeed I was informed by countless, yet elder physicians, that interns and residents "lived" in hospitals, at least those training in certain specialities, like mine.

I don't doubt this.

Nor do I doubt that equally horrendous events occurred in earlier years.

The Chiefs of training were God like creatures then (some still are), shattering what was medically sanctioned, and developing what is modern surgery today.

They created you, directed your life, your future. They were in charge, not only of your body, but that which made you, you. Your needs where secondary to their whims. At all times, it was understood, should you fail them, you have failed your patient. This was a constant, and for most, unbearable burden. Remaining candidates truly were dedicated, driven, intense.

Physicians have been known as caring people for millenniums. Society rewards those amongst us, who would choose such path, with honor (you call your physician, Doctor Jones, you never address a carpenter, as Carpenter Jones) respect, and usually a significant income.

I have not always seen a "correlation" between these benefits and an individual's performance. We are all human with human frailties and weaknesses.

What amazes me nevertheless, is finding the occasional exceptionally bright individual doing very, very stupid things, atrocious decisions, even committing fraud. Why, when a person has everything, would they act so badly?

Can we identify these individuals before they have a very prolonged and expensive training? Indeed, how does the average layman choose a physician? Being Board certified is a good start. Careful of marketing.

Admittedly, even I would have a difficult time finding another type specialist for my family. Surgical Nurses/techs may know when a surgeon is clumsy, but they don't see patients afterwards, so that physicians judgement may be terrible in selecting cases. They wouldn't know.

I have seen many a technically proficient surgeon do repeatedly unnecessary surgeries, or wrong type, despite performing technically a marvelous job.

Sometimes it's a popularity contest. Marketing, especially self marketing, is quite useful in that regards, as is publishing papers.

Of course, we select our presidents that way. When was the last time we saw a candidate for this high office demonstrate their knowledge of Geography, Economics, or political science by way of "written exam"? Doesn't happen.

Being good looking, a smooth talker, and smiling does help.
Same with physicians.
Conversely, the Physician with no bedside manners may be thought of as

having great surgical talent. (with such an attitude, he must be great).

There are so many caveats in evaluating your surgeons, a separate book would be necessary to delve into them all.

Consider the surgeon who can perform a complex operation with acumen, but repetitively performs "lesser surgeries" with little interest, even disdain. Do you want this person to be your surgeon?

For instance, a surgeon who operates on the spine must be a good carpenter, but not to recognize that prerequisite would be neglectful. One such surgeon told me at the beginning of his career, how much he disliked the majority of the procedures he performed.

How does that work?

It gets a little more complex then, in selecting one… just because aunt Bessie said he helped her, and she recommends them.

Ever think of why your local physician sends you to a particular specialist?

Is this the best one for the job? Was he friends with that surgeon in medical school? Are they cousins?

Does that surgeon refer many patients back to your Primary Care physician, for General exams, lab work?   I have seen all these abuses.

Sorry, I've seen a lot, and most referrals would indeed, seem appropriate. But it happens. And worse.

In any case, the following, while upsetting to some, may educate the Lay person a little, as to the extremes that certain intense specialties demand in recruiting the younger generations.

Please bear with me, as we proceed to negotiate my road to the present.

CHAPTER 4   FANCY AND NOT SO FANCY PEOPLE

There obviously was a mistake.

I was accepted to the most prestigious University Hospital (large city) as Intern.

The stories got better, and much different.

A Downtown hospital with awesome reputation in a very livable area.

I was assigned an Apartment on the first floor with 17 ft ceilings, and one bedroom.

There was a small wall for a kitchen, one bathroom and a refrigerator in the entrance hall, far from the kitchen. Curious, but all still very cool.

I bought JBL speakers with a Sansui receiver.

The walls were solid concrete in this old structure (Razed the year we left for a new Hotel).

Hospital patients included VIPs and their wives, both of industry and politics, Titans of sports, a slew of obese women with gallbladder disease and great addresses, strippers, mafia, other physicians from different hospitals, and the you's and me's.

And, I received tips. Expensive Champagne, 50 yard tickets (now this would probably be frowned upon) and more, were gifted from patients who were pleased with my assistance in their care.

By then, I was convinced I could be a spectacular Neurosurgeon.

Sitting at the Nursing station, doing chart rounds about midnight one day, a staff physician turned to me, and probably out of boredom, asked my future plans.
"I plan on going on to a Neurosurgery residency after my Internship," I answered.
He smiled. "I was a neurosurgical resident for Harvey Cushing."
The Neurosurgeon of a Millennium, most famous, known for his temper and talent.

What?
I turned from my tasks, to find him gathering up his charts, to place back in their bins.

"Please go on," I replied, knowing he was a well respected internist.
"Well." he answered.
The day after I got married, I was called to the chief's office.
He continued. Cushing turned to him and asked, why?
Interesting, because that year, I myself, was asked by a Neurosurgery Chairman when interviewing, "Why did I get married?" I had just married a few months earlier.

What did you answer? I asked.
Well, I told him that my wife was a nurse in the same hospital. She knew I "lived there" and I could assure him, this would have absolutely no effect on my work.
He paused, then said, "Harvey told me to pack my bags, I was out of there, now."

He turned walking slowly away. I watched him until he disappeared into the elevator.

I think I sat there frozen for a good ten minutes, some nurse interrupting, about a patient.

So there was a famous general surgeon, at the same hospital, who did very large and lengthy surgeries. Everyone, it seemed wanted a (Surgeon's name) incision from Fancy town. I became his intern.

Because he was known for operating throughout the wee hours, the hospital made a ruling, no cases that were elective, could begin after 3 PM.

Play the game they say, and so it went. Midsize cases early in the day, then smaller cases so he would be ready go with the longest, at 3 PM.

On large bellies, which he frequently operated on, he would make a 16 inch incision, followed often by a cross incision of about 18+ inches.

Knowing how long it would take to close these operating wounds gave the Intern a chance to ponder his mortality.

The surgeon would always make 5, not the usual 3 ties to each knot, and would close with many more knots than average. Thus, a closure could take several hours at the end of a long case.

One evening after operating on a patient for a number of hours, he said quietly (as he always spoke), "we need to do a Whipple's here", adding on another 6 hours for that case.

The other intern holding a large retractor, swooned.

Are you okay? asked the attentive surgeon.

"Just my Diabetes I suspect." replied the young man.

Well played, I thought. Whether or not he had that condition,

his portion of labor would fall unto me.

How did this old guy (probably then in his late 50s) manage to keep

on going? Has he no bladder?

I was realizing that although I was now an intern at a most reputable hospital,

(even making a good $5000 a year) opportunities to become a Neurosurgeon,

seemed lessening.

There was, simply, no time to study.

Every month or so, was a new rotation.

Despite this, I looked forward to one of the most challenging rotations, that

of the Emergency room. It would give me practical experience.

Also, it promised me, many new stories.

Almost daily.

We were on 24, off 24 hours. I would see up to 112 patients each day by myself.

There was only one physician for the biggest ER downtown, and those 2 months,

it was me. Some were very brief encounters, others longer, but still averaging

about 10 minutes per pt.

The nurses had great fun with me. I liked them a lot, nevertheless.

The first week I came there, I saw an old black man for constipation.

I asked how long he had this, and was told 60 years.

The nurses were giggling.

Apparently the responsible family member worked downtown, but lived far away.

There was simply no other way to care for the grandfather, so they dropped

him off in the Emergency room every week, at least once. The nurses understood, and let him stay there. He wasn't a bother. He was family.
The man would just sit in a chair for 8 hours, and occasionally talk with other patients, or their family members.
No harm, no foul.

Sometimes the joke was played on us all. Then we were less tolerant.
An executive with diamond cufflinks, gold rings and Rolex, found that side when he interrupted a huge crush of patients one evening, with the complaint of urgent constipation.
You're kidding? I asked the RN. That's what he said, turning away, after handing me the chart.
This can't be happening, I mused.

Two possible heart attacks, a large laceration, an undiagnosed fever, possible pneumonia, and these were just the patients in the exam rooms, not the overfilled waiting area.
Seriously? I asked. How long have you been constipated. He answered, about 4 hours. After a diligent search for other conditions he might be confusing, and basic psychiatric analysis, I concluded he was simply "a jerk".
The nurses looked to me for guidance.

Admittedly I was a triage physician for all the important cases, with consultants on the available, as soon as the patient had my initial workup complete.
But still, 112 patients!
I would go home and collapse, sleep 4 hours, then wake up, and later try to sleep another 4 just prior to my next 24 hour shift.

So I'm looking at a beautifully tailored gentleman in luxury clothes, telling me he can't have an elective bowel movement.

This probably was not the lowest I sunk as a physician, but it certainly was fun. I told the nurses to take away all his clothes, excluding underwear.

Give him an oral medication to induce a bowel movement, and an extra strong suppository. Then walk away. We all agreed, to share the cleanup.
Loud voices were heard after an hour or so, from his room.
Only a sink was available to him, there was no commode.
I don't think he was happy. But I got no admonition from the Hospital Administration, and the ER Nurses and staff supported this response to "ER abuse."

Then there was the "You can't win" situation, as you really can't.
A young boy age about 9, was brought by his frantic mother, after allegedly being hit in the head with a bat. He checked out okay, but pretended he was not responsive. I thought a lesson was in order, so I reached down when his mother didn't watch, and squeezed his testicles.
Holy cow! He shot up wide awake looking for an explanation for mom, who was not privy to my gentle assault.
Another exam done in front of mom, found a very cooperative young lad, having no reason being in the ER. There was no real history of head injury, no loss of consciousness, only what his friends thought "might" have happened.

I took mom aside.

Young boy sitting up on gurney, eyeing me suspiciously.

Standing with mom about 20 feet away, and speaking in hushed tones, I offered my opinion.

I explained that he was a normal appearing young boy who had no evidence for head injury, including any scalp contusion. And perhaps everyone panicked a little, out of concern he was truly unconscious.
I thought we could discharge him with neurological precautions.
I explained this, as we both smiled towards the youngster, and agreed, with the plan of action.

As I was concluding what I thought was a superlative counseling to an obviously confused mom, a large suction bottle (in those days glass) spontaneously fell off the wall, for no reason, crashing on his head rendering our little lad, now truly dazed !

Admission to Neuro for observation. Enough said.
Can't ever write a book about this stuff. Who would believe?

Good thing about the ER though, I got to take care of Playboy bunnies.
They often had several jobs. In addition to waitressing, some were airline Stewardesses, and some were also, we would say, with the "the service" industry.

Because of this connection, however, I was valued as a source for pretty girls to attend intern parties. They saw it as an opportunity. The Interns saw it as, "Hey, works for us" !

My wife saw it as a bad joke (still does).

So it was not surprising one day when I was called to make a "house call" for an ailing hottie.
I was in the ER shift, and no could do. But I had a friend who just might.
A most grateful friend, who promised me fealty to end of time, when the offer was mentioned. Everyone was happy, no?

"Best laid plans." Again?? Come on.
So why the anger? His belligerence the next time I saw him a few days later, was palpable.
A nurse took me aside.
"When he was doing a "house call" there was a raid on that domicile, and he was brought in for questioning." His wife was not very understanding.
Ooooh.

Remember this was the Age of Aquarius, Viet Nam was heating up, and considering my obvious run of luck, I expected I would be called up to our Armed services. I went to our local Navy recruitment agency with the intention to enlist, in what was called the "Berry Plan." I would be allowed to finish my specialty training as long as I promised to then serve 2 years in the Navy, as that type physician.

Not many Navy facilities deep in the jungles of Nam, I reasoned.
The officer sat me down, and asked me to read the chart on the wall.
I am extremely myopic (nearsighted) without glasses, and replied, I saw no definite chart without them. He laughed and said I could never be accepted into the Navy,

with such vision.

Okay with me.

I got up, but he looked at some paper again, and asked what I did.

I'm a physician, applying for the Berry plan.

So breathe.

What?

Just breathe.

Like this, I asked somewhat comically.

You passed, he answered, still sorting some papers, not smiling.

You'll get your notice in the mail.

Next.

Well, that was interesting.

We're in the Navy dear. Nice, she replied.

The remaining time at this University hospital was spent in various surgical rotations.

Stories did not slow down.

I particularly enraged a soon-to-be divorced general surgeon, by refusing to pass a Foley catheter on one surgical patient, until the he was asleep. There simply was no reason to do this awake, when it could be done comfortably, in a few minutes. I expected continued trouble from this otherwise fine young surgeon. Happened, he responded well to the challenge and logic.

We became "Bros".

Go figure.

Then some senate investigating committee came to town, and one Mafioso took a section of the top floor of the hospital, "to recuperate."
Turns out, I was a "good kid" and could I pass him that bottle of Chianti?
This was before the godfather movies, and he spoke just like Marlon Brando, in the film.

Getting on, there was this gentleman, whose family name is on products we know and use today. "His jet, from L.A. will be landing at 10 PM, please meet him at the front door of the hospital". I was given a suitcase, beautifully handcrafted, and full of medication in gorgeous matching bottles. I mean filled!

On helping him unpack, he earnestly asked, if he needed more pills. I didn't even have time to do a history and physical on him, yet. But, he was asking someone who (he must have known) had no knowledge of his medical case. Befuddling.
And he is a CEO?

Experiences. Some very strange. Others, kinda nice.
Like when a world famous, baseball player (you know the name) was made to wait 6 hours in the ER because I had so many really serious cases t see first.
Surprised again!
He was kind, and not angry, that his fame brought him "no" medical priority.
I was very impressed. Humbled.
Shouldn't prejudge.

My next rotation was also surgical, and here is where I found my true calling as a medical detective. Some of the immaturity I so relished, began losing its attraction.

I wondered about why a stripper whose art form was making her mammaries swing with tassels in opposite direction, demurred for a breast exam.

A lady with a totally see through mesh dress (that's all) appeared as a family member, for an urgent admission. Where did she receive the call?

But it was a lady with a car accident that really got me to thinking about my "job."

On X ray. (No MRIs or even CAT scan then) she had a fractured transverse process in the lumbar spine, age undetermined. But she complained of severe pain in that location. A kidney injury could have occurred as well. Admitted at night time to my service, I examined her and noted a peculiar affect (facial expression). I made little of that, finding no other significant injury, or suspicion of one. Early the next morning I was called to see her because she was now passing blood in her urine. A good deal of blood.

I consulted with the staff who ordered further urological tests, which was negative. That afternoon she suddenly spiked a temperature of 106 Degrees. What's going on? She looks good, otherwise. The nurses where told to take her Vital signs much more frequently, and call if any changes.

Going by her room in the middle of the following night, a nurse motioned for me to have a word. I can't be sure, she commented, but I thought I saw her place the thermometer (in those days, glass) on the radiator.

I looked in on her. A repeat temperature (new thermometer) was normal.

But more blood than ever found in her urine cup.

This was puzzling.

Turning in, I awoke shortly thereafter, with an answer.

I immediately called our blood bank, to see if any blood products where missing.

None where.

The following day, still a temperature randomly, and more blood.

I sat down with the patient and went over everything I might have missed.

Plan was to let further events declare themselves, per attending urologist.

I wasn't satisfied.

Unwilling to give up my fanciful idea of blood source, I contacted another Hospital which joined ours, through tunnels.

Why yes, they exclaimed! We are missing a unit of whole blood.

What's going on?

A search of the room, when the patient went away for further "urine tests," found the plastic container, still labeled, with some blood, in the back of one drawer.

Now that was amazing. A Munchausen Syndrome, in our back yard!

I began to talk to patients. Still, I wanted to see illnesses, understand

their toll, the treatment available at the time, and especially, do procedures.
I was informed one night of a man with internal hemorrhaging. It couldn't be controlled. He would die soon, his BP falling. In a private room, door opened, I looked in. There he was, breathing fast, barely conscious.
His thoughts? Did he have any at that moment?

And other random observations.
How can a heart surgeon put a valve in backwards?
Oh yeah, he was the same cardiac specialist who was a chain smoker.
Clearly our lives are complex, and not necessarily logical.

Some people you can argue fought hard to get their disease.
Others became innocent bystanders of fate's cruel hand.
Children and babies not spared.
I began to "feel," at the wrong time. This was a distraction.
I didn't want to see some of the horrors any more.
And how do Pediatric specialists, Oncologists especially, survive?
God bless them, for it. But I began to get emotionally involved, and I didn't need that.

It was thrilling, hard work, and damaging at the same time.
As a mere technician, few patients really wanted to interface, in any case.
I wasn't "their doctor." I was the one that came down in the middle of the night to restart an IV, start a Foley catheter, or other menial tasks.
I did make note, however, that most people were very nice, and rarely cruel, when sick, though there were exceptions.

Without necessarily being predictable.   Remember mention of the earlier case of a world class Sports figure. That guy was amazing. He talked to me. Likewise some very Fancy people, also looked my way, at times to be friendly.   There appeared no direct relationship with social standing, or severity of illness. Most puzzling.

I learned which diseases I feared most. Surprisingly this was advanced COPD, ALS, and for whatever reason, metastatic Melanoma.
I planned on picking a cardiac arrhythmia as the easiest exit, from this dimension.

Now Interns were a tight group, because of the 24/7 schedule I suppose. Most of those impressed me as quite elegant. They were gifted care givers, worth emulating. The attending Medical staff was also awesome. Two steps above the Charity hospital group. Having said that, one could only wonder how they would act, if placed in a similar situation, as opposed to their upscale offices, operating rooms with air conditioning, even a hospital physician dining room (that at the time had a selection of wines).
Didn't really matter. It was, what it was.
All in all, the Medical staff was respectful, the Nurses all bright and cheerful.

However, there were holes or gaps at times, that raised questions about the administration's attitudes (generally judged very supportive).

My Orthopedic "elective" was in winter. At night, the sleep room had a portable air conditioning unit, with large gaps about the window.
Basically, room air was close to outside air temperature.

A small very hot radiator tried desperately to keep the room above freezing. I would cuddle next to this, located against the bed.
But every few minutes my backside would repetitively ignite, after touching this inferno.

I looked around. I found a dangling bare 60 watt light bulb for illumination, and replaced it with a 100 watt from another empty room, and stuffed in as many towels as I could about the AC unit, all to no avail.
I was pissed.

Desperate, I went into an adjoining area, got some plaster of Paris and put a "cast" over the entire window. At last, 66 degrees!
No one complained.

My time was getting short, and I looked to joining a Neurosurgery Residency Program. Final rotations included ENT, Ophthalmology, and Neurology.

All were pleasant experiences, not physically challenging.

Chapter. 5 WORLD CLASS IN A UNIVERSITY TOWN

I contemplated my next step, in a small midwestern University town. This would be where a Neurosurgical resident would learn some more Neurology. My wife immediately was offered a position there as an RN. My plan then was to take a full Neurology Residency, not just a Neurosurgical rotation elective. This was "suggested" by my Chief, as a way to mature.

Coming from a downtown apartment luxury area, to a University surrounded by farm land was, well, wonderful. I had not lost my direction, it was clarified.
But this was a time to relax a little, and learn how to study!
Drawbacks were no fine restaurants, (actually anything close to that) distance from our parents, and friends.
We didn't have the money or desire for "shopping". So that was a non-issue.

On a side note, all our close friends we made there, have looked us up, after decades, and we have reunited. Bucket list, I know.

As for the program, it was recognized as one of the better Clinical Neurology training areas in the country.
We were happy.

We didn't need much, except for ourselves and Neurology texts.

One senior resident recommended a Gilroy and Meyers textbook of Neurology,

then Plum and Posner's on coma.

I was ecstatic!

And more. I actually was learning "how" to learn.

Patients were enjoyable, though sometimes, suspicious of a non-local.

Having said this, the University hospital had Physicians training from all

parts of the world, and friends included people from South Africa to

South America.

So the Neurology program was calm.

Sort of, but leave it to me to find excitement.

Only the first year residents took call, sleeping at night in the hospital.

We slept most nights without interruption in a dank basement,

sheets always moist.

Could be worse. It was only every fourth or fifth night for one year.

I learned EEG, EMG and a then had a further rotation in Psychiatry.

It was at the latter time, out of the blue, I concluded that gay people were born that way, and not trained or perverted into such life style. It was normal for them.

Admittedly, I am more organically oriented, than many. Even if this status was environmentally produced, I argued, it would be accompanied by hormone or other body chemistry, not just regulated by mere circumstance or indoctrination, which I would point out, still are reflected In body chemistry. Maybe we haven't heard the last on this analysis, so I stand ready to listen. But I have held these views since 1970. Haven't seen any scientific literature yet to dissuade me.

While met with some disbelief, most of my peers, even at the time, respected that opinion as one possibility, however, unlikely.

Still working through what "normal" means in psychiatry, however.

Their VA facility was unfortunately, like many of the other VA hospitals.
The Neurology head there, was counter to our University Neurology Chief who was, I believe, a teetotaler. Whenever I entered the former's office, all lights were out, the blinds on the small windows closed, and usually accompanied by the sound of a desk drawer snapping shut, with bottles clanking, and the whiff of alcohol.

The patients, Veterans all, accepted their lot.

However one amusing situation, should be mentioned.
I found a patient living there for more than a year, with no hospital records suggesting an explanation, let alone documenting his stay.
The saying "good enough for government work" struck home.

Back to the University proper, I asked my Neurosurgical peers to call me, when they had an emergency. I had a camera, I used to record slides of arteriograms, patients photos, and surgeries (no HIPPA then).

One particularly troublesome case was a man who attempted suicide with a shotgun. I was told it was a terrible idea. Apparently, if aimed at the face, it often "bucks" causing the gun to violently "redirect".

The consequences were no jaw, no nose, no eyes, but brain intact, and alive.

Well, in this case (witnessed) it was more terrible, if possible. The remainder of his mouth constantly filled with blood, and intubation was impossible.
He choked to death on his own blood. Autopsy confirmed no brain injury.

In a similar vein, another patient was seen with a severe facial injury from removing a tire rim, tire already inflated.
This equally destructive force from the rim exploded into his face, compressing what were eyes, eye sockets and nose into oblivion, fortunately and still unbelievably, sparing intrusion into the skull and brain.
Blind but wiser. Also, serious nasal reconstruction needed.

Contemplating some of my Neurology patients, I got to be amazed even more, if possible.

Hard working farmers could cut off a finger and continue working the rest of the day. The sun was another matter.

In those days, a hat was survival. Except for one older gentleman.
Every time he put on a hat, he would pass out!

Our suspicions were confirmed, by performing an arteriogram.
He had total occlusion of most major arteries inside the skull (supplying his brain).
Instead, collateral circulation about his scalp, went "through his skull" providing blood to that vital organ.
These alone prevented a stroke, or even death… unless he put a hat on.

Such simple activity, would occlude the blood supply to his brain, and threaten his life. Best solution, a different type of hat, or shade.

Technology wasn't awesome then, but logic was.

Now one of my best stories from those years, was a patient who had Multiple Sclerosis. This was a very pleasant middle aged lady, who developed some temporary weakness in an extremity or two because of that diagnosis.
After a course of steroids, she responded quickly, so that after a week or so in the hospital, she was much improved.

I was chief resident at that time, and usually made rounds with 8 or 9 other nurses, junior residents, and medical students.
The patient and I had enjoyed a close relationship, and I told her I believed she could be discharged, earlier that day. I summarized her case for the audience, and proceeded with my previously discussed plans.

I asked the Junior resident to take over rounds for the group, seeing next, her roommate, as I took her to a waiting room, which was empty. I would write the discharge orders and final arrangements for follow up, etc.
Entering the room, a TV was quietly on, but of no bother, and the staff was told to temporarily keep the door closed, until this short matter was completed.

We sat down on a couch, and she immediately began thanking me for her care.
I replied, it was a pleasure to do so.
Beginning to write the discharge note, she interrupted.

"You know, I consider you a friend, as well as a physician, and I trust you. So I would like you to know how I got this condition."
I stopped writing the final discharge order.

I felt a little twinge of what might be coming. I wasn't disappointed.

Well, she began, "when the Martians landed, they sprinkled me with Pixie dust."

I peered into her eyes to determine her veracity.

This was no patient-doctor joke.

Go on, I implored, quietly tearing up my last note and discharge orders.

"Sure," she softly replied.

"I have electrical powers at times, and can control things with my mind."

"I see." I answered cautiously. Would you be willing to discuss this phenomena further with a specialist, that might have better knowledge of such powers, I asked?

"Well, I certainly trust your recommendations," she replied.

"Who would that be"? she asked?

I suppose a psychiatrist might be the best option for such an experience, I suggested, relying on her trust and naïveté.

"If you say so," she smiled, "I would be happy to explain these things, to whoever, you think best."

By this time, I had already wrote for a Psych consult.

Well then, let's go to the Nursing station to see what needs to be done for such consultation (expecting a transfer to said service, would be indicated).

Her family would be informed that she wished to pursue this avenue upon their pending arrival.

We got up and walked to the door, which I opened for her.

Upon passing me, a TV next to this door suddenly made a very loud electrical sound, went off, sounding like a muffled explosion (tube type).

She turned to me, my mouth agasp, and said, "See"?

I suggested maybe further discussion with the family and discharge with a community Psychiatric evaluation, at that point.

"Whatever you think". she added.

Won't forget this one, I contemplated.

The mind is a powerful tool.

This was further demonstrated when obvious pseudo seizures in patients would be abruptly terminated by passing an NG tube half way down.

Psychiatry, did have its foundation in Neurology, I was reminded.

I also have concluded in writing these memories, that life is random.

Totally unexpected things happen. Patients intentionally, and more often unintentionally, can confuse the diagnosis, the treatment, even the prognosis. And they, are us.

Then there was the poignant.

A patient having metastatic carcinoma from the lungs throughout his body, enjoyed nothing more than rolling his own cigarettes for the day, sitting on the edge of his hospital bed, when doing so.

He smoked constantly and his room was filled with the fumes.

A reminder. Smoking was allowed in the hospital then (cigarettes even sold in hospitals for another 20 years).

This man who had months to live paused, during one exam.
He turned, knowing his diagnosis and prognosis.
Looked me in the eye, and asked, Doctor, do you think I should stop smoking?
It was thought provoking, even at the time.

But I knew what must be answered.
If you enjoy them, why not?
He smiled. We both understood the logic.

This Regional midwestern Medical Center had many world renowned physicians.
Some specialities like Urology, particularly eminent.
The speciality was dominated by a chief, a gifted tyrant who treated his residents as "men that could take it". Don't recall any women in Urology training there.

So my friend, who was a senior Urology resident, ready to fly on his own in a few months, took certain privileges. Like asking his chief when assisting him in surgery, did he "want the knots cut too long, or too short."
Of course, there was a limit tolerated.

In the middle of one night (read that as about 2 or 3 AM) my friend was doing chart rounds, and catching up on the work from the day before.
He told me of the footsteps coming far away in the dark corridor, getting louder and louder.

What's the Chief doing here at this hour, recognizing his gait?

Impossible. Surgery will start in a few hours, and this would limit any sleep options. Like "not."

He turned knowing the Nursing station was in a dead end corridor, with no back staircase. "I hid in a closet," he confided to me.
"I could see him through the louvres of the door."
Exhausted and hot in that closed space, he remained focused on fantasies of a wonderfully supportive bed, how good it would feel.

After half an hour the Chief got up, shoving charts aside.
He began to walk off, then stopped.
Then turned back, and knocked on the closet door.
"Okay to come out now, Glenn." he boomed.

My friend didn't, until the Chief could be heard, trailing far off .

Embarrassed yes, regretful, maybe. Sorry for a wasting a half an hour standing in tight quarters with a broom? Oh Yeah!

He was a gentle creature who excelled in his training.
I still remember being shocked when I heard he died a short time after going into the practice of his dreams, from a brain tumor.
Even sadder, he was a General Physician in Texas before his Urology residency.
Both he and his wife had saved for years to raise a family, during the coming additional training. Really not sure there is a lesson there.
Tragedy chooses randomly.

Fortunately we made a number of very good friends in that little town.
Their unique experiences added to our growth as much as any major

Metropolis could. So it was a welcome pause.

Peace and Fun times? Yep.

Sitting in a ground floor apartment with some friends, and sharing a drink or two, I remember someone observing that "something just hopped past us". Uh, Huh.

Well there it is again!
A bunny. A small bunny!
Unreal. No one's pet, for sure.
We followed him to a bedroom, where we would liberate him from a self imposed predicament. (Could have been a "she").

A plan was devised..
I would kneel down in my new bell bottoms pants, and catch him, so gently.
If for any reason he would escape from my intended assistance, the wife and our friends behind me would be back up, for what would be a very controlled situation..

He then would be returned to the farmland, which surrounded our apartments. Or, at least outside.

Didn't want to scare the little critter who obviously thought there was stew in our eyes, not a needed friend.
Had to take care not to panic our tiny fella.

He came out from beneath the bed. At last, no escape!
Best laid plans.

Of course, even a small puff of a creature, can be elusive.

And very fast. Right past me it flew, suddenly realizing, I had reinforcements,

retreating into the safety of my bell bottom trousers.

Holly Moly! Now that was not considered.

After extirpating myself and God's little creature, we both concluded,

it was a most unpleasant experience, not to be repeated.

But, it is one to retell, as you get older. So here I am.

Chapter 6   THINGS CHANGE RAPIDLY

Prior to the end of my Neurology Residency, I started looking for a Neurosurgical one to follow. The last 6 months of Neurology training could be an elective, which I chose as Neurosurgery. Two birds with one stone, getting credit twice in that fashion.

I was pleased with my training in Neurology, but needed to return to my true love, Neurosurgery. And, I wanted something different.

So, I interviewed at several locations.
One picked in part, for its convenience and familiarity, another opposite home base, highly recognized.

It was winter. I drove through a blinding snowstorm for 8 hours, only to find that my interview with the Neurosurgical Chief was cancelled because he couldn't get out of the driveway, "with all that snow".
Undaunted, I drove another 8 hours to the next location for a second, now first, interview. It was also a prestigious facility, maybe a little more so. The Chief there, interviewed my wife as well. Basically telling her, she would be a widow for the next 6 years. That was understood. My wife was very supportive of all my endeavors.

I even interviewed at a southern Medical center of recognized international fame, because of an historical event.

The Department chief there took me about proudly introducing me to his present residents. He even boasted that a few months ago, he actually drove to an airport, to stop his Chief resident's wife, from leaving him. Something to do with being a resident's widow, never seeing her husband.

Flying round the campus everyone seemed quite competent and very impressive. He then asked, if I would need lunch. I jumped at the opportunity, hoping to learn more about him, and his role in history.

He turned a few feet later, and entered a small area of the hospital that sold carry out food items. He asked, if I liked eggs? Curious, I replied yes. Wherein, he purchased one hard boiled egg for me, and suggested we proceed with the schedule, motioning to the exit.

What did I expect?

I eventually chose bachelor number one, hoping some winter storm might block my driveway, like it did his. I didn't make it past summer.

Turns out the Navy was serious about me serving as a Neurologist when my training was complete. And, they really didn't like the concept of further specialization.

After only six months into a Neurosurgical residency, gotta pack up again.

My reintroduction to Neurosurgery was interesting.

Expecting a camaraderie of sorts with the staff (I was now a fully trained neurologist) I found myself lower than a first year resident in Neurology. I guess you can't just "expect", respect. You have to earn it, especially with this group.

My brief six month further training, would end shortly, most noted for my constant muscle pain, especial in the upper back. Neurosurgeons, turned out, needed to be physically, not just mentally endowed.

I did see some interesting cases, even in that brief time, including an intern who just sledded down a hill into a tree after new snow fall, only to stand up, with a neck that was fractured, severing his spinal cord.
He didn't survive.

But soon, I was to start the obligation.

Chapter 7.   A Call to Duty

Happily, I got to choose between three location options, by the Navy. I listed them in order of preference, I suppose this was out of politeness, since I was assigned one, I had not picked… on the east coast.
Well, no matter.

In fact, it did matter. I loved their selection.
I was able to do EMGS and EEG's, moonlighting for extra income,
and maintained the rank of Lieutenant Commander.
My salary was awesome, compared to my past engagements.
And a new venue !

As a Naval Neurologist, the chances where slim for deployment anywhere near Viet Nam, still boiling over, and the experience was fantastic.

I got to board a nuclear attack submarine (the Captain had the same rank as this young nerd), commandeer a jeep to position, at the end of a runway, as an F 14 roared past (photos came out well, but bad idea considering our jeep type vehicle almost flipped over with the force of the "Afterburner"), and toured up and down the east coast from Newport Rhode Island, down to the new Disney World. There were some inconveniences. But the adventure well worth it.

I saw another type of patient, young, usually healthy.

Not all were however.

Early on, a young man presented with symptoms that befuddled his local physicians.

He had problems with remembering at times, a little difficulty swallowing and some problems with coordination. At the time the history was obtained in a small office, followed by a neurological exam on a rudimentary bench.

CAT scans where only done at Bethesda for special cases, and this was well before MRIs were invented.

I observed a brief twitching of some muscles, as he rested his bare forearms on my desk opposite me.

I looked at him, and took a guess.

Are you a Chamorro, I asked?

No ! He screamed.

And kept on screaming.

My bad. Got the fatal diagnosis in the first few seconds.

Unfortunately the patient was well aware of this condition from his home in Guam.

There definitely had to be a better way of presenting my thoughts, at least in the first few seconds of an interview. I almost cried.

How could I have been so careless.

It took some time for him to gain his composure.

Multiple corpsman by then had arrived, to check on the commotion.

I sat next to him.

Dismissing the others I explained, nothing was definite.

Neither he, nor I, believed this.

The degenerative condition in Guam, was Amyotrophic Lateral Sclerosis-Parkinsonism-Dementia syndrome, later referred to as Lytico-bodig disease.
It was the leading cause of death in Guam between 1945 and 1956.
The consumption of bats was hypothesized responsible for this disease.
I was positively brilliant, and overwhelmingly stupid.

There was a disconnect. Terrible way to learn.
I comforted myself in concluding he would still have to be told,
and no matter how I tried, I couldn't conceive of a way that was truly gentle.
Gentler, maybe.

During those days, even as a Neurologist, on some weekends, we had to work in a Navy Emergency Room. Can you imagine a Psychiatrist sewing up a laceration? That was the joke, knowing a Neurologist might be equally incompetent in the latest treatment for a myocardial infarction (heart attack).

But I was a little shocked to find that myself and a fellow Neurologist would be assigned as GMOs (General medical officers) for a shakedown cruise
(just 5 days) on an aircraft carrier.
Just awesome, I thought! My fellow Neurologist from New York City,
who was perhaps the closest friend of mine in the Navy, shuddered.
"We're gonna die!" I think, was his response.

In all fairness to him, I did write up a medical report noting his history of occasional severe Migraine. We both knew that wasn't going to fly.
So trying to restrain my unbridled enthusiasm in front of him, we were

shown to a cabin with a bunkbed.

A fuchsia colored vertical pipe by the pillow said "JP-8 Fuel" (or something like that). There were no windows, of course.

My friend took the upper bunk, immediately grabbing a handful of various colored pills. "What are they?" I asked.

Flippantly, he replied, "Don't know, don't care."

Actually, I think he rather enjoyed the time on the voyage,

It was no cruise ship, but physicians were regarded by everyone, including the Captain, as almost Royalty.

Being tall, I had to be careful though, noting everyone over 6 feet, was said to eventually receive a concussion, from overlying pipes, and machinery.

This particular ship was in Viet Nam previously, and had a massive explosion with significant loss of life. Safety was everywhere, but it was a warship. That was certain.

At night, having free reign of the ship, I walked out on the massive elevator deck, now at the level where planes were stored. A thin single cable separated me from the ocean below, no handrail here. And, no one around, save for my reluctant friend.

Realty check there. I stepped back.

Brought my camera, and got unbelievable photos of planes taking off, Captains bridge, etc. The brass must have thought we were, insane. We certainly kept them amused. But, that was not our function on board.

Waking up to a Philippine service man, providing us breakfast, on what appeared to be a silver tray, and wondering if we went "down the rabbit hole", our assignment was to provide general medical care to a couple thousand young men.

Great guys, highly motivated, was our general consensus.
Some issues did present. Including an "Anniversary Reaction" in an emotionally distraught man, who lost his wife a year previous.
And the usual coughs and colds.

Rummaging through papers in my metal desk draw, I found evidence once more, that this was a warship. It had inherent dangers not only to others, but even the crew. Older men would talk about losing a guy or two on every long cruise, just rolling off into the ocean, when Carriers were not air-conditioned, and men slept on the long narrow outsides. Again, no women on ship at that time. Suppose it could have happened.

About a dozen papers in a folder, mostly Greek to me, with the plethora of acronyms, abbreviations, titles, and identifying numbers, all lie in the pencil drawer of my metal desk.
But the reality, was one technical Naval personnel working on a radar, beyond the recommended time allotted, crossed 2 wires and received, like 2 billion volts of electricity. Little to do, but pronounce him charcoal.

Alright, I wasn't going to go there. Exploring the ship seemed more pleasant, even half safe, when off duty.
Why, I could scope the accompanying rooms to ours where fighter pilots decorated their doors with Eagles or lions, tearing things apart. (These guys all seemed to

look like Robert Redford, and were inseparable).

No serious injuries were seen fortunately, though I could understand how things could go from routine and boring to real dangerous in a heartbeat.
Don't know if they still have alarm-to-quarters "X, Y, Z, and operation Chopsticks". Ask an old Navy man about these (scare the crap out of you, especially the last).
But, it was a pleasure serving those men. dry land still welcomed.

Now at that time, I still fancied myself the budding Neurosurgeon, so I would connect as best possible with the Neurosurgeons, especially those my age, to discuss cases, even socially. And, I volunteered to help them in surgery if needed, after hours.

They had a slightly different lifestyle. On weekends they were shuttled by Helicopter a hundred miles plus, to a Marine base to see consultations.
They were at risk to being sent off, to "hot spots" for Emergency Neurosurgical care in field. They certainly earned their wings (uh fins, I guess, since we're Navy).

They got the respect they deserved.
One Marine transferred unconscious, found himself waking with a Neurosurgical Chief knuckling his chest, and asking him his name.

First thing our young marine sees, coming awake, is a 4 striped epaulette, Naval Captain.
"I'm nothing but a shit, sir"
God bless these guys.

Sometimes an injury had humorous results.

Notable was a condition known as Saturday night Palsy, where a young Naval man imbibed too much alcohol, and fell deeply asleep on a chair, or with something in his armpit. Also known as a radial nerve palsy, it caused inability to extend the wrist.

These would generally recover fully in 6 to 8 weeks.

The trauma of not being able to properly salute a senior office during this time, might take longer.

We did see a number of hereditary neurological conditions, some rare and interesting. But many were simple Migraines, or other benign conditions.

However, even benign conditions could have major consequences.

A sailor with "night terrors" running across the ship in his sleep, or one with Narcolepsy (suddenly falling asleep) for instance, let alone a patient with uncontrolled seizures, all would limit their abilities to function as required.

And just like that, a wonderfully peaceful two years passed.

About the only stress was taking my Neurology written Boards in Washington D.C.

"Aced" those.

And now back to the Midwest.

But before we leave, there were a few days…

Is There A Doctor In The House?

We heard that in old movies right?

So there were ten or so days in 1973, that I was that doctor.

Well, not exactly "house".

The first occurred during a stadium show of Lippizaner horses, where these beautiful animals did highly controlled stylized jumps and other intricate movements. The audience was quite large (as I remember, in the thousands) awed with the feats performed, when two of them collided.

Wow! That wasn't planned.

One rider fell to the stadium floor, momentarily unconscious.

So the call "Is there a doctor in the house"? really blasted over the loudspeakers. I jumped into the arena, and ran to the fallen victim. This had occurred on the side opposite to where my wife and I were seated. So by the time I arrived, another man closer, was already conversing with a groggy, and certainly stunned performer.

I identified myself as a Neurologist. The other attending gentleman looked up at me and commented he too was a physician, but he "forgot his stethoscope." What? Who says such a thing? He promptly left the scene. I shook my head and went back addressing our fallen patient.

After clearing said horseman of any serious injury. (mild concussion), and accompanying him off the arena, I heard again the loudspeaker, now announcing that all was well, and that a "young physician" was caring for him.
Why young? It was true at the time, but I felt somewhat marginalized by that comment, like, it was "the best we could do under such sort notice."

Wasn't two days later, when at a stop light, a motorcycle was sideswiped in front of me, by a car. The guy slid over a hundred feet, on asphalt. Fortunate for him, despite the balmy weather, he had on thick boots and an impressive leather outfit. I assumed the worst, but was amazed he had only a few cuts and scraps, nothing serious.

I'm going somewhere with this.

Same week I found myself on a plane ready for takeoff, at O'hare airport. A lady unbuckled her seatbelt and fell to the floor of the airplane, moaning and verbally unresponsive.

Examining her took a few minutes, history obtained by a helpful relative accompanying her. Apparently the lady appreciated some of her symptoms prior to the flight, and had already consumed some orange juice, for what was apparently, not her only such spell. She became progressively more responsive, assuring me all would be well, "it always responds to orange juice."

While prior episodes of similar nature was comforting, a new event of different cause, could not be entirely excluded, and I went through my usual questioning, and exam.

Above me stood an anxious gentleman (beside most passengers straining for a better look) either the Captain or copilot, don't recall. Apparently we had finished taxiing, and were ready for take-off, behind us, a bazillion planes and far more passengers aboard them, wondering what was the problem?

Should we abort? He asked, like it was a life and death decision. Could have been, I suppose.

But no, I believe she will be Okay. Headphone on, he conversed further with the Tower, and we were back on our way to the east coast.

Needless to say, my eyes were on this lady the entire flight, hoping I didn't miss anything. All was well.

Finally a couple days after that, I found myself in a crowded church, near the front, seated next to the aisle. The service already was in progress, when a young girl could be heard walking up from the back, stopping next to me, then passing out. Once more of benign origin… but really?

Have to have some business cards made up.

Alright, seriously, I felt so vulnerable during these times, without proper equipment to address, what might have been serious events. Outside of controlling bleeding, or preventing spinal injury in transit, there was little more possible (barring CPR). A diagnosis without available treatment, is as good as no diagnosis.

But, I Digress.

Chapter. 8   A. Final Plunge

We picked up my folks and drove back to the University Hospitals to continue my Neurosurgical residency.

I was told by my Chief that because I was gone, there would be a reshuffling of Residents, and I would have another half year added to my training.

This was not in our verbal agreement upon leaving to serve in the Navy.

I came down and explained my disappointment to the rest of the family.

My dad, said no!

What?

He continued, "go up and tell him that was not your agreement, and this is not acceptable."

Not a comfortable conversation. But I started with that comment, and got back an "okay" from the Chief.

Six months of my life, was that negotiable?

SERIOUSLY ILL PATIENTS

Now began in earnest, the final training in Neurosurgery.

Sometimes there were just silly adjustments.

Like the time, now (again) the junior resident, I was told if I needed

to call in a senior man, I was also that person, since I was a fully trained neurologist.

Obviously need to perform major brain surgery, an exception.

Or, since we also served a VA hospital one mile away, I would be responsible

at night for starting IVs, Foley catheters, etc for the Neurosurgical floor.

I had no car (this was at home with my wife who traveled for her new Nursing career).

A bus may not even be running at those hours, and certainly would not be

a direct connection, or I could walk railroad tracks in sub zero temperature,

back and forth in the middle of the night (2 miles total). Hopefully no emergency

would occur during this jog back to the main hospital.

An alternative, was to be REALLY nice to some other resident, in a different

Specialty, who stayed "there" nights, and would assume these tasks for me.

Guess which one I chose?

Let's start off with being on call some years, up to 125 to 135 hours a week.

And by being on call, I meant doing work, and staying at the hospital.

Do the math and calculate sleep hours.

In fact, I was happy to get 2 out of the 3 basic human functions in a day.

The first, probably doesn't come to mind immediately.

Everyone has to pee !

Yes that minute or less to micturate was valuable, even if a nurse was pounding

at the door, asking for some orders. Sleep was also needed. Catch some here,

some there, it could enable survival. Seldom an hour straight, but we could always hope. Finally, food. Give me a break.

After the last Residency in Neurosurgery, I rarely ate breakfast or lunch,
Including liquids until night time, for about 35 yers.
Watch out at night time, however. This isn't grazing, more like a feeding
frenzy.

In my last year as Senior resident (jumping ahead) I asked my Chief, for
one night off a month. Everyone was impressed with my audacity.
He agreed! Well, didn't usually pan out, as promised.

It got so bad that I was still doing work at 3 AM planned for the day,
before. Patients complained.
We would make Neurosurgery rounds with everyone at 6:30 AM.
They were being awakened up a couple before, just so I could finish up
daily tasks.
My chief said, "this had to stop."
Please tell me how? I asked. He never did get back to me on that one.

My Junior Resident, once didn't sleep for 72 hours. He asked our chief,
at that point, "what would happen, if I collapsed?"
This occurred after our Saturday conference, noting we had a full Neurosurgery
clinic, as usual, following that.

I was there. I heard the reply. "Don't worry, you won't"!

I told him I would cover for him, and to get a couple hours sleep, in the on call room.

Less than half an hour later, my Chief paged me.

He asked where my junior was? "He's here seeing patients with me", I replied.

Should I get him out of an exam room?

"No that's fine", was the reply.

I'd like to think he changed his mind.

(Muffled laugh).

Our life was Neurosurgery, which is to say taking care of frequently very sick patients.

For this, I would gladly have endured the above.

Difficult cases from around the state came to our tertiary care center.

The saddest, and most hard to accept by the family, would have been a young girl with major head injury, or inoperable brain tumor. They needed extra support. Which isn't to say a young man following a motorcycle accident, left brain dead, couldn't have a similar grieving family at times.

I still remember a torn father, asking over and over again, why a helmet his son wore could not protect him, since he was only doing 25 mph? We could at times, just sit there with them. Let them speak how wonderful he was as a child, how everyone loved him. This cut into us, as well.

Then that night, be called to see another young man paralyzed following a bicycle accident, heavily inebriated. I asked him why he rode in his condition, on such hills, and traffic. His reply, with a smirk "I was too drunk to walk".

Can't make this stuff up.

A judges son diving head first into a lake, was left quadriplegic.

Spring is especially dangerous, I concluded, up North.

Young men seemed prone to diving into uncharted territory, head first.

One local Neurosurgeon actually brought up placing all young men during Spring, on steroids, thought to be of some help prophylactically in spinal cord trauma.

He may have been not entirely serious, but point made.

I thought of another ward, a few years earlier at the downtown University Hospital. Changing a Foley catheter, I overheard one paraplegic bitterly complaining of his lot to another, who was quadriplegic.

The latter rebuffed him, crying out, "you dumb SOB, at least you could pull yourself up to that window"….pointing to one open, being 10 stories up.

I couldn't imagine my life being a quad. Most horrific existence?

Their parents would eventually tire out, or die caring for them.

They would be in some back room somewhere, becoming lonelier and lonelier, more desperate, a scream for help, knowing none could.

How do some, remain sane, even optimistic, yes productive?

What internal strength do they find, especially since most were young men, who really had yet to live?

I was always reverent. Yes, that's the word, to use when about such patients.

Explaining my admiration, at their adaptation, and encouraging them.

But, my God!

Fortunately, my chosen specialty did not always have sad stories as it may appear. One Saturday Clinic, found a lady in her 50s being assisted by her husband. She was barely walking. Her extremely awkward, slow pace, was impaired further by her elderly husband who had a severe limp.
She was incontinent of urine, and had significant recent memory problems. Both feared the probable diagnosis of Alzheimers disease suggested by family members. Enter the new wonder machine, a CAT scan.
It demonstrated large ventricles (hollow cavities that make the spinal fluid) causing pressure on her surrounding brain.
This condition was just described a few years earlier. It's called Normal Pressure Hydrocephalus.

A shunt with a valve was passed from the brain cavity to the belly to absorb the trapped fluid. She went home a few days later. But when she returned for a two week follow up, it was her, helping her husband walk. And she did this in high heels! Memory good, yep, and no further incontinence of urine.

Another interesting case was an unlucky gentleman, who hit a deer with his car, doing about 60 mph. Not good for the car, not good or the deer, and not good for my patient who received a horn in the brain, when the deer crashed through his windshield.

The horn was cut flush with the skin by a local Emergency medical team. He did fairly well after a craniotomy to remove another three inches of horn which stuck deep into the brain, although he had some speech deficits unfortunately, since the horn hit him in the left temporal area, which relates to that function.

I'll later tell you about two almost identical stories, that occurred in private practice. You might better understand why I chose this specialty, outside of the obvious physical and mental challenges.

I should add, not all Neurosurgeons are created equal. That was obvious from the start. By now, I had the passion and the tools to be the best, in what I did. Not everyone apparently, had that need.

One Neurosurgeon a few years earlier was run out of town when it was proven he did "sham" operations. He went to another state and started over again. Two other Neurosurgeons I worked with had limited skills. We were there (the Neurosurgical residents) to protect patients from those buffoons, and for the most part succeeded.

But, my gosh to see a fine Neurosurgeon operate, was like Opera and Ballet together. Masterful strokes, intuitive, logical, cautious when needed, and most of all guided by sound judgement.

Some of the best were in private practice. We rotated under their tutelage, to get as broad as possible an experience. All of those, save one, were exceptionally gifted.

Everyone's favorite appeared to be the senior Neurosurgeon, who (I believe it was in the mid 1960s) was said to have done a clipping of a Vein of Galen Aneurysm "Live" on TV! Won't go into the details as to the diagnosis, or surgery, outside of say it is challenging surgery, especially for the time.

My personal hero.

It was also said, he won a television award for this documentary. I'm sure his patient was even more pleased, having had an excellent result. It seemed everyone In the hospital was familiar with that story.

I would frequently ask his opinion about cases I was to perform for other Neurosurgeons. He would reply, "well, I would do this approach, but with your limited experience, may I suggest what probably would be safer for you to perform, with the same results." Never felt insulted. He was on the patient's side at all times.

Best I seen. Newer techniques arrived, and, I personally in practice, performed more complex surgeries, than he ever dreamed of doing.

But this "takes the man out of his time".

There simply was no equal to him.

Saw him decades later, in another country, where he retired raising sheep there, for another 20 years.

He was still "the man".

Back at the University hospital rotation, even a semi quiet night, could develop into mayhem. One Neurosurgical resident, earlier in the day performed a routine lumbar discectomy, removing pressure on the Sciatic nerve, causing his pain, and some paralysis.

The patient initially did quite well.

Then about midnight when I was there on call, he started having increasing back pain. An attentive Nurse informed me she was worried, adding he had a precipitous drop in blood pressure. I listened with my stethoscope to his back, and heard a bruit. This is a sound made when an artery is narrowed or injured.

I called the vascular surgeon team, who immediately performed an Arteriogram, confirming my suspicion. A very small piece of major artery was removed when an instrument went too deep inside the disc space.
I followed him to surgery. It was a mess.

Blood pressure by then was critically low, so IV fluids, followed by blood when available, was pushed at a rapid rate. One of the surgeons exclaimed after an hour, "this must be the artery here". The anatomy was so distorted, the surgeon found it difficult to even identify the mischievous tear.
You will be happy to know that patient did great!

Also, totally appreciate that nurse who was on her toes that night.

There were still the spectacular injuries, like a farmer who, for whatever reason fell on a high voltage electrical wire, landing on his neck. Most of his neck appeared burnt off. Where were the carotid arteries in all that black debris?
And since he laid on his back of the neck, one vertebral artery was plainly seen, exposed to air, despite all the charred damage. How to handle? He was awake, and unbelievably, moving all extremities.

The tissues were basically non existent for repair.
Our staff elected observation, understanding probable progression of his

wounds. It did progress. The vertebral artery to the back of the brain blew one night, and he exsanguinated. On the other hand, it probably would have happened to the unlucky surgeon if intervention was attempted. Still, both patient I'm sure, and surgeon felt totally helpless to the inevitable.

Within six months of that patient, I was in a VA rotation which shared the floor with vascular patients. One young man had cancer of the neck, and his surgeon told me further repair was impossible. The Nurses had standing orders to give him Morphine when this artery would explode.
I was there when it happened. Blood shot on the wall, and it seemed like the entire floor, about his bed, filled with his blood… in seconds. It was over quickly.
Things to ponder. A lot.
Why him, were there any options the surgeon did not explore, and endless second guesses? He was not my patient.
That didn't make it any easier.

The situation was desperate on the Neurosurgical side as well…for a different reason. An Oriental Neurosurgeon who lacked empathy, ran the show. Remember these Veterans at the time, where mainly from WWII. They couldn't tell the difference between Japanese, Chinese, or other Oriental ethnic group. This created endless friction, that the residents tried to bridge. This wasn't easy. It gave added stress to managing most patients at that institution.

But there were simple joys at times, and endless shaking of our heads at humanity's foibles.

One not so happy event, was a middle aged alcoholic, that was being treated for another condition. He wished to sign out, but there was a terrible winter storm, and any travel was not wise. He insisted on leaving. I personally told him, his plans were not adequate, and there was a good chance he wouldn't make it to his destination a hundred or more miles away. He was found frozen to death the next day, by some highway Patrolmen.

Not taking medical advice, or in this case weather advice, has consequences.

Sometimes not.

Two men shared a room at the end of the unit. Both had a fractured cervical spine. One was in his twenties. One in his nineties.

Now in those days we immobilized the neck by sometimes placing a metal halo ring screwed to the skull at four points, vertical rods connecting to a body cast, applied with the patient sitting. Both had this device on. Of course, the younger man would heal faster, and with greater certainty, noting they had similar fractures. So he was allowed discharge sooner. A few weeks later he came for a follow up visit. The entire device, cast, screws in the head etc., were all removed. What happened? I asked Who removed these? That was too early in my opinion.

"I did," he replied.

He saw me contemplating a response, and answered further.

"You know, in the garage, I worked at".

Faith smiles on flowers. He did well.

As for the man in his nineties, a far more interesting follow up occurred.

Again, in those days, the VA hospitals would allow a "furlough" for some patients. Basically a weekend off, to be spent at home (or wherever). After a month in the hospital, he seemed ready. He could ambulate by himself, feed himself, and in general, take care of hygiene matters adequately.

I had between forty to fifty patients, as I recall, on the neurosurgical floor and additional patients on other services, that had neurological problems. This would mean basic rounds to be completed before the start of surgery at 0700. Track shoes were advised.

So one Monday morning, I was coming up the stairs, and who should I see, our ninety (plus) old man standing in his hospital room door waving vigorously at me. "Can I have a word doctor" he shouted, as I zoomed past.

Not wanting to speak in the hallway, and frankly being pressed for time, I motioned down the corridor, to come to my office. He wasn't the fastest sprinter in that outfit (cast), his age also a factor.

I hardly looked up, when he entered.

"How can I help?" I asked, barely recognizing this fine gentleman. He understood my work load, and was sympathetic. Didn't even sit down, standing in the entrance. "I have a question," he voiced softly. "Ok, I answered."

"You know I had a furlough this last week".
"Of course. Did it go well, any problems?"
"Well, just one".

"I looked up. What happened?" I asked.

"Well, I was with my wife, and I couldn't."

"You couldn't what?" I replied, still rustling papers

"You know, with my wife," he answered.

Slightly frustrated at having to devote another small portion of my brain to this endeavor, I sighed, and glanced up.

"Can you be more specific?" I asked.

"I couldn't have relations with my wife," he spoke softer.

Now he had my attention. A smile crossed my face.

"You mean sexual?"

"Yes," he answered.

"Could you before this accident?" I asked, amused.

"Yeah," was his response.

Now here's were it gets a little "gamey". I knew I had a connection with this patient for some time. So in part because of that, and my still impeding need to finish rounds and chart notes, I took the liberty to blurt out, "You know at your age, I would be happy to pee with it!"

He smiled. Standing, still waiting for an answer.

"Well, I sighed, if you could before, I see no reason, neurologically, why you couldn't now." He smiled. He knew, I was sincere.

He then ambled out of the room, we both kept that smile the rest of the day.

Chapter 9   The End Is Not the End

Sitting in an on call/sleep room, some time later, now almost a senior resident, with the man who presently was the senior resident, on the couch /night bed. He was breathing hard. He looked at me somewhat desperately, and said, "I don't think I'm going to make it"!
He had another half year before completion of the program.
What did he mean?

Actually my first thought was, "If he was gone, the work load would surely kill me".

Usually we rotated once every three nights, frequently once every two, and sometimes two nights straight, if the others were sick or took their limited vacation days (One week per year).
To be clear, when "on call" that meant a minimum of 36 hours straight, so two nights straight, meant three days being in hospital (and potentially no sleep about 60 hours. While that wasn't likely, it was likely, we wouldn't get four unInterrupted hours a night.   The couch/bed would remain a promise.

One gone leaves two, to share that already crazy workload.
My mind was swirling.

Sure you can !

He better, my survival depends on him!

I described his glorious future, telling him of the paradise to follow.

He would move south, buy a fancy car, work maybe 80 hours a week, and find that beautiful suburban house, maybe with a pool.   Hang on, just a little longer. He knew he had no choice. Maybe venting helped a little.

I could certainly understand his feelings, getting close to that point, myself.

Thank God, he buckled up, caught his breath, and decided to plow through.

He understood, there was no alternative (save the unthinkable).

Then came the phone call.

Destiny is a cruel master.

Both sitting once more, in that same small room, a couple weeks later, busy organizing the day and following night duties, with the occasional odor of burning body parts, from our small window.

Sorry for that last point, but how do you think these are discarded by a hospital? Apparently a vent for this, was nearby.

It was the Chief wanting to speak to the senior resident.

Come to my office !

The conversation was to the point, my friend returning to the small room in twenty, or so minutes.

He wasn't tearful this time. He was totally ashen.

He spoke sitting inches from me, looking straight ahead.

In a monotone voice, he began, "The Chief says I have to do an additional six months Residency."

There was a pause. Both of us examining our options.

"He said because a resident (we both knew who he was referring to) went to the Armed services for two years, there was a disruption in the way residents would graduate."

We both sat there for a few minutes.

Then he got up quietly and left.

I honestly didn't know if he would "off himself".

He didn't.

There were many desperate cases. Maybe that effected how we viewed our own hardships in comparison. Wasn't even close. The focus was totally on them.

I already alluded to parts of my own senior residency.

It was a blur.

I do remember being allowed to perform increasingly complex cases.

One particular type I hoped to perform, was called an STA to MCA anastomosis.

For patients who had diminished blood flow to the Brain, and were susceptible to a stroke, one option might be taking the large skin artery (you can palpate this by your temple) making a large hole in the skull and attaching it to an artery on the brain.

10- O or smaller suture was utilized. So fine was this (less than human hair) that different techniques needed to be mastered in the lab, before performing that type of surgery.

For instance, we all have a physiological tremor.

At high magnification and with this type of surgery, it could make performing the operation difficult, not possible…if you did't use techniques to stabilize the instrument held.

An arm rest, and more importantly a hand rest, were essential.

Water was your enemy. A drop of it would catch the fine suture like a magnet. And if the nurse accidentally dropped the suture passing it to you, good luck on finding it on the drapes. Well, I was only too excited to learn about the technique, even though I never did such cases until private practice.

This just might be very helpful for a select group of patients. I began to study about it. Explaining to my mother on the telephone about this bypass surgery, may have been more challenging.

She and dad had waited 10 years after my medical school graduation, through my training and Navy stint, to brag on their son. I think she had the vaguest notion of what a Neurologist did, but now her son was going to learn how to do "bypass surgery"!

Her only question was, as a well informed Reader's Digest fan, how do you stop the heart?

No mom. I'm talking about bypass on the brain.

"Oh," she answered, somewhat disappointed. "But you could do bypass on the heart, if you wanted to"?

My wife who was on the extension line, quickly interrupted. She would definitely not be a widow for a third residency program.

No mom !

Going on....

Chapter. 10   A New Beginning, New Risks

January is not a bad time to move south from the north, snow covered roads aside. After shoveling the roof once more (didn't want that to collapse after we left) we now had two cars, both packed and ready to go, and a walkie-talkie for communication range within 75 feet. We had no CB radio, and certainly no cell phone then.

I chose a location to practice first, because of its natural beauty, where I wanted to live, and one day retire. Then a hospital I thought was forward thinking, and finally a neurosurgical partner.

I was incredibly confident, having turned down an offer in a large Southern city for ten times (10 x) the amount salary offered, which I declined. The pittance of economic renumeration I accepted, would surely be "offset" by later significant increases, and that is were I wanted to call home.

In the next couple of years, I would move my folks next door, my wife's folks a few blocks away, and her other daughter and her three children all into the same area. I even moved one of my professors who taught me neurosurgery, down south. Unfortunately my partner at the time, believed my former professor joining us, might side against him, with me on certain issues, and he wouldn't agree for him to join our group.

In the years to come, I would move a number of other neurosurgeons to my new home city. All in all, transition successful.

It was a very pleasant surprise, to find out a year later, that the Oral boards (final Neurosurgical examination) would be held in my city, meaning no travel was necessary. On leaving for the exam, my wife wished me the best of luck, reminding me (and I quote) "Our entire future, depends on this".

That certainly broke the tension.

But, I did my best to undo even this, unintended blessing.

One of my examiners, a Nationally renowned Neurosurgeon, welcomed me into his exam room, his desk prepared with items for my evaluation. Casually, he tamped some tobacco into his pipe, and out of courtesy, asked, if I would mind him smoking. I replied yes, I would.

What self destructive demon, still resided in my soul?

We both paused briefly. I, contemplating if my future was smoked in a glib reply (pun intended), and the examiner contemplating his own reaction.

He smiled devilishly, and I briefly assumed this was out of respect for such audacity. We will never know. What happened next however, drew serious question as to, not only the wisdom of my brashness, but that examiner's love affair with his pipe.

The smile was more than prolonged, lasting through his gathering of previously placed questions and items on the desk, placing them slowly in an attache, and still smiling, bringing forth a dozen or so rigid cardboard "Visual fields" performed on patients with various brain and ophthalmic lesions.

These were exams of real patients who had lost part of their vision, which would have localized the offending lesion, through such testing. They were not the simple "bi-temporal hemianopsia" variety. (Vision loss caused by a pituitary tumor on the optic chasm).

I don't recall my reaction, at the time. These were challenging items for any neurosurgeon. Fortunately, and I do mean very fortunately, as in, I had no reason to expect salvation at this point, I was already a fully trained Neurologist as well, with some interest, during a prior residency, in visual field testing. Even then, I doubt I answered all correctly.

Courtesy remained. And I left puzzled, if my response might have indeed, resulted in near catastrophe.

Wristwatch check, wallet check, keys check, common sense… well, must have left that on the dresser, this morning.

Strange, I didn't feel at much risk being an outsider in private practice. But I was. The gentleman I joined, while competent, didn't have the social or legal clout of a big group, and I was in the highest risk specialty for malpractice lawsuits.

These attorneys soon noticed a new kid on the block, and some lawsuits did arrive. I couldn't understand it, then. How could I be sued for ordering a test on a patient that wasn't even mine?
Or, because my partner did something, they believed warranted a lawsuit, I was included in the complaint.

Best one, deserves some elaboration.

A young man was transferred from another large hospital with a severe headache and confusion. That facility, despite their size, did not have a Neurosurgeon on staff. On examining him, I determined he had a subarachnoid hemorrhage from a brain aneurysm. Surgery was performed immediately, for a ruptured anterior communicating aneurysm, successfully. He woke up with the only residual, a slight clumsiness of his left hand, not from the surgery, but spasm of the vessels that frequently occurs from this type of hemorrhage.

A wonderful result. The patient was happy.
A few months later, I received the claim. It was from the most formidable plaintiff attorney at the time, with my name, up top. I called my malpractice Carrier immediately and explained, that I had a good relationship with the patient, and he knew I saved his life. I told them I wanted to call the patient personally and discuss the lawsuit. He was horrified!

I eventually told him I was going to write a letter to the patient, asking why he believed I committed any wrong. My malpractice attorney very reluctantly agreed, informing me, the consequences were all mine.

Within days I got a response. The patient, a nice, but real country boy, wasn't told I was to be included in the suit, he wrote. He felt ashamed that I was so humiliated, and already spent a day in his attorney's office to cancel my name from the claim.

But his attorney didn't show up. Not to worry, "if he couldn't stop this action against me", he assured me, he would "testify on my behalf"!
Unreal. Totally.
   Oh, still got the letter!

And, I have taken care of his relatives, who he refers, decades later, even though he no longer lives In our state.

After the first few years, all that nonsense settled down, and in the last 30 years of practice I only had one further lawsuit, but this one is worth mentioning.

A morbidly obese pleasant man, had lumbar spinal stenosis. This is narrowing of the spinal canal, causing severe pain, and at times paralysis. After reviewing the risks with him, I performed surgery successfully alleviating all his pre operative pain. Three days later however, he said an incident occurred, and he had a tremendous increase of sciatic pain again, but no other symptoms.

I told him to go the Emergency of my hospital. The ER physician examined him

and noted he was neurologically intact, but in significant discomfort. We agreed on admission, and I would see him in the morning. Neurological checks were ordered. During the night, he developed paralysis in both legs, and bladder.
I was not informed.

The next morning I was shocked to see his condition and quickly determined he had a Cauda equina syndrome, bringing him to surgery, within about 14 hours after admission. Post op, all motor paralysis resolved, but he was left, at least for an indefinite future, with a neurogenic bladder, occasionally having to self catheterize. He would at times soil himself, if his stools were loose.

The Plaintiff attorney confided with mine, that I would not be included in the lawsuit, "If" I would agree to testify against my hospital and nurses, who performed below a standard of care.
My attorneys "strongly advised against such action". (They were very smart).

It went to court, my first and last time.
Opening statement by the plaintiff attorney described me as caring and an excellent surgeon (or similar words). I looked to my attorneys.
What's going on? They motioned for me to remain quiet. Noting across the table were the nurses who saw the neurological changes on my patient, recorded them, but did not call me.

Each of the 3 nurses (ER Nurse transferring patient, night nurse, and AM Nurse) all responded, that they "thought I was notified", and "should have been", one even said, she "Hoped I was".
Didn't their attorney prepare them?

Then I was called to testify. After a brief response to several appropriate questions, including that I would have moved quicker if called that night, (even though that probably would not have changed the results) their attorney said I was quite cooperative, and they would dismiss me from the lawsuit.

A multitude of attorneys called out from all points of the room, demanding "Side bar" with the judge. He determined this action was appropriate, and recess. declared. The jurors left the courtroom.

Apparently, the Nurses' attorneys then wished to question me, and cast some blame in another direction.

The patient and I gave each other a big bear hug in court.
I was sorry for what he went through, and I thought he was sorry for the 18 months I spent preparing for that day.

The case eventually turned out much more bizarre then that, but I would leave this vignette, commenting that the neurosurgeon who was to testify against me, previously had an identical lawsuit (management of a caudal equina syndrome), And, on reviewing his disposition from his own case, I observed that he gave the opposite opinion, when he was "the defendant."

Recently, another Neurosurgeon called me about that Individual, who apparently is just "a gun for hire".

I'm glad I had one such experience, but I wouldn't want to do this again, Nor would I wish this on a young Neurosurgeon. Such attacks, are taken very personal, if you know you did what was right for the patient, including tireless dedication, and making his or her problem, the number one priority in your life.

It effects your entire family, as well, usually lasting more than a year, or two. Unlike in business, this is not just "the cost of doing something".

I was told by our National organization at one point, that on average, every neurosurgeon should expect such a lawsuit every four years. I guess I was very fortunate in my career.

But, we're just at the beginning of this journey.

Chapter 11.   Foolishness, to much Gravity

Admittedly, I am very proud of my profession and its soldiers.

They are true warriors against disease, trauma, tumors and much much more, often under very burdensome conditions.

The brain and spine are the ultimate frontier, at least on earth.

Don't venture into this arena, if you expect an easy ride.

Enough levity,

Occasionally some people just play the system.

Heck, we all probably do, sometime or another.

So when a young man age 24 told me that his back still hurt after a work related injury, it was not unusual. Sometimes this can happen even with normal Imaging afterwards. His following remark caught my attention.

"I think I should be on disability" because I worked "all my life".

You're 24! If injured permanently, fine. But don't expect sympathy because you worked a few years.

This was followed up within months, by a mother who brought her 16 year old daughter for evaluation of back strain from a work related issue.

Mom told me she thought her daughter should be on permanent disability.

Whoa! Is that even possible with Workmen's compensation?

But then there are those who really deserve such consideration, that's obvious.

A twist on that, was an grandma raising her grandchildren and receiving benefits because of a severe tremor in the upper extremities. She couldn't even use her dominant hand to feed herself.

I was doing deep brain stimulators (DBS), and felt reasonably certain I could control that issue for her. While there was some risks, she decided against the surgery, for fear that she would lose disability benefits, if "cured". She couldn't afford to return to work "and still be there to raise all her grandchildren".

Who wouldn't be sympathetic to that dilemma?

A few years into my practice, my partner and I decided to find another Neurosurgeon to be in our group. We were able to entice to our area a talented man, who had as much testosterone, as myself. It didn't end well. But, I would have to share any blame for that.

During his brief stay with us, an interesting case presented.
A lady was evaluated for a vascular malformation in the brainstem.
This is most challenging of brain areas to consider any surgery, because of extreme risks to the patient. We were young, confident and worried that another hemorrhage could kill her. I asked him what he thought? He answered, "Let's do it". I wasn't so sure.
It was a judgement call, one that placed the patient's life for extreme risks,

either way.

I decided at that time, to pass. I had a better idea.

I would send her to a neurosurgeon in Canada who was the first to operate in this area. He was internationally recognized, as one of the few with big enough Cojones to attempt such surgery.

She agreed to go.

A few weeks later I received a phone call from this eminent surgeon,
He commented, he would also pass, adding If he did the surgery, he "would kill her".
His suggestion, was watchful follow up, only.

She returned and thanked me for, my sending her to this awesome surgeon, and understood the consequences of his, I'm sure, gently placed remarks.

I then saw her in an outlying clinic for a year or two, after which time, she was lost to follow up. I feared the worst.
Half a dozen years later she reappeared in this clinic, with an amazing tale.
She had moved out of state, and now came back.
I was overjoyed to see her.
And she looked great!

I sat down with my old friend, and asked her if she had any problems where she lived?
Just once, she added.
Tell me about it, I replied.

Well, they thought I had another brain hemorrhage, so a neurosurgeon was consulted. This was in one of America's finest Medical Centers.
What happened? I asked with more than a little curiosity.
They recommended surgery. They told me it was high risk, but they thought we had a good chance of fixing the problem.
She had my full attention.

I was admitted to the hospital, and taken to the surgery area, where the Neurosurgeon arrived and reviewed again what was to follow. Adding he had the utmost confidence In his team, and appreciated the confidence I had in him.

She continued, "I told him, I had confidence in all the neurosurgeons that treated me," including the one in her home state (that would be me), and the one in Canada.

"Who saw you in Canada?" he asked, with surprising alarm.
She mentioned the trophy Neurosurgeon's name and she reported him, visibly shaken.

And he advised against this surgery? Her present neurosurgeon queried further.
Yes, she replied. He thought it far too dangerous a procedure.

Then she looked at me, and in a more serious voice, said, "he sat down and told me the surgery was off." I was sent home that day.

It was obvious even to this fine lady, what had transpired.

If something went wrong (and it quite possibly could) he would have disagreed with the world's preeminent specialist on this matter.
For all we know, he might have had some training with him.
Bad situation for him.
Turned out it was good for the patient.
We both shook our heads, and smiled. See you next year.

That little rural clinic through the years, brought me more phenomenal cases than I could have imagined.

One such was a patient with a very large benign tumor.
I later took my OR Nurse who assisted with this case, to a national Neurosurgical meeting. A similar tumor was presented, as truly challenging.
Ours was twice that size.

It extended from the Right frontal area to the occiput, then to the cerebellum. (There was even a similar tumor on the opposite side.) In other words, from the forehead to the back of the head, even a component on the left side.
It required an ENT surgeon to assist in removing the Ear bone and help close.
We didn't attempt to remove the tumor, in its entirety, that would be too dangerous. As it happened, she had a rocky first few days post op. But, eventually she did fine. We smiled, when that presenter described how huge an undertaking, was this most unique case.

Another fascinating situation, was a lady who had cancer, replacing most of the neck bones. I removed all the vertebral bodies (from C2 to C7) replacing the bones with a single bar of methyl methacrylate (plastic cement), screws in the top and bottom vertebra to hold it in position.

This was successful enough, that she lived years longer, despite the cancer having spread to other areas of the body.   Amazing !

And, she remained neurologically intact, during those follow up years.

Chapter 12.   Sometimes Medical Progress Takes Its Time.

Two such examples follow.

As a Neurology resident, I was able to take a trip to Europe where my wife and I skied France and Switzerland. On the return leg, we scheduled a visit to Queen's Square hospital in England. This was about 1970-71. The trip was amazing in so many ways. We flew on an early 747 and saw the new Concord airplane on the Tarmac at Orly airport, Paris, learned to drive stick shift in the Alps, and was given a warm reception at the hospital where as a guest, I was invited to make rounds with them.

One patient had Huntington's Chorea. I was particularly interested in this disease because I had a large population at my midwestern hospital.
How are you treating this? I asked.
With Nitoman they replied.   You most likely know this as tetrabenazine.
No I didn't.

But on coming back home I presented the experience to my staff professors
The drug was not available in the United States.
Well, about 40 years later I saw an article, discussing this as a new medicine in America, to treat Huntington's chorea. To the best of my knowledge,

it took that long to bring it across the big pond.

While a resident about to return to Neurosurgery, I had no capability in starting a grant proposal, for research on the drug, at the time.

Look this up and be astounded.

Progress delayed again, when as a young neurosurgeon, because of my early experiences in private practice, I became more reticent to introduce new procedures.

I did start "microscopic" operations on the spine. One was called microdiskectomy. To my knowledge, I was the first in my part of the country, to perform these routinely.

Patients were able to be discharged the next day, and shortly after introducing the procedure, the same day. It was many years before this was accepted as a reasonable alternative, in my state. In fact, one established Neurosurgeon in the community complained to the chief of Surgery, and his hospital (where I also performed surgeries) that the operating microscope added additional time for a procedure, since It had to be "balanced" before many cases (true, but this took a couple of minutes) and added to the time of surgeries (false, and proven).

He just didn't like the operating microscope, not even using it for his intracranial aneurysm surgeries, preferring surgical loupes (simple magnifying lenses on eyeglasses) instead. He wasn't trained with this tool, and firmly resisted.
What, can I say?

I was challenged and responded. Eventually this would be the Gold standard, for most cases. Until then, some believed the Operating microscope was simply, not essential.

I was aware nevertheless, that other Neurosurgeons were observing my work, and became more cautious in introducing new techniques, such as measuring intracranial pressure, following severe head trauma (now also accepted).

About 1979 I also had the opportunity to see an unfortunate young lady who just delivered a baby. She had a compression fracture from metastatic cancer. I still remember this clearly. I made a tiny incision over that vertebra, cleaned out the cancer, which could be readily removed and used a syringe to fill the bone cavity with Methyl methacrylate (a cement like substance). I did a number of such case before I stopped doing these, noting no one else in the state was performing such surgery.

About 15+ years later the procedure became a hit, now called Kyphoplasty, or Vertebroplasty, using a large trochar (Large bore needle) to deliver the plastic, instead of a small incision, Vindicated again!

On another note, patients (us) can be quite amusing.
But sometimes, we can amuse back.

Some years ago I operated on a Russian scientist for a spine problem. He was extremely pleased with his results, and gifted me a small bottle of Vodka and caviar. Then came the good part. He moved close to my face, and asked if I would like to know a secret?
"Sure?" I replied, hesitantly.

"I be Russian Nuclear engineer on our submarines years past, following your submarines underwater."

I laughed. "That's not half as funny, as you know".

My wife's Uncle (also Russian) was "our nuclear engineer for some submarine tours checking out U.S.A. systems." He lived near Pittsburgh, a trained nuclear physicist.

Two Russians underwater. Made you think.

Each of our countries have problems. Politicians will endlessly debate them.

I would like to see a President of ours develop a committee to study how to "improve" our relations. One for each major country.

Small steps. Don't have to be naive, just try to develop a common bond !

CHAPTER. 13. A Practice Rollercoaster

Then, there were some very scary cases.

One involved a gentleman with an A-V fistula. Blood went from a very high pressure system to a low pressure one without necessary capillaries. Humungous veins developed, from what was an extra cranial arterial supply. Multiple rope like vessels pulsated on his scalp feeding this monster.

The last thing we wanted to do was operate.

His condition deteriorated with some intracranial hemorrhage.

I could see this man getting a haircut and bleeding-out on the barber chair, if one of those were nicked.

The vessels passed through openings in the skull, the size of finger holes, going deep inside a midline structure called the Falx, where the fistula called home.

Taking one scalp arterial supply might result in other vessels stepping up to replace them within 24 hours. And these might be deeper and much more dangerous to approach. Placing glue or plugs inside these huge pipes also was ruled out at the time. This was in the 1980s.

I remember the operating rooms, the details of this case even today.

The evening "before" the main AM surgery, I tied off all the extracranial (scalp) vessels. That following morning was "tight sphincter," as I hoped I didn't miss any of the "outside supply" for this creature…or, they didn't reconstitute quickly from inside brain vessels. If that happened, we would be the Barber Chair, and he would have seconds, before he lost most of his blood.

We turned the bone flap with a saw. No hemorrhaging. Then lifted it from the canvas like membrane (called dura) below.

The skull bone looked like Swiss cheese.
The case wasn't over yet. We had to go deep between the hemispheres of the brain to find this little devil. A single aneurysm clip on it, and he was out of danger. Whew!

Then there was the absurd.
I received a letter from the Medical Board in my state, asking me to respond to a patient's complaint.
I did a Cervical laminectomy on her, from which she did well.
All pain and paralysis resolved. No unusual issue noted at any time, either pre, or post op.

Her complaint written, stated that after surgery, men followed her around with shotguns in their car, and (this will get your attention) "Every time I have sex, I can see the future". What the folks on Wall street, could do with that talent.

On another level of reality. Not the slightest clue through the entire time, she was in my (admittedly brief) care.

And a number of patient memories were "happy-sad."

An elderly lady with terminal cancer, screamed continuously because of uncontrollable pain, disturbing other patients on her floor.
This went on day and night.

I was consulted to assist in any neurosurgical recommendation for pain control. Narcotics did not touch her, and more could not be given without worrying about her having a respiratory arrest.
The Cancer was everywhere. Pain was not in just one locality.

Her oncologist told me she just had days to live, but seemed unlikely that either the nursing staff or other patients on floor could tolerate any more. They looked desperately for answer from everyone. Any ideas at all how to make this time easier for her?
I sat down by her bedside. Tears rolled down from her eyes, and she grabbed my hand.

"I know I'm dying doctor. But I can't stand the pain. How much longer do I have to bear this, please tell me?"
I paused, contemplating, how I should reply. Other physicians had been reluctant to offer her a definitive response.
I thought what I would want to hear, lying there?
I then said "about 5 days"

She was shocked. "Five" she repeated?
"Yes, I believe so."
She thanked me, and closed her eyes.

The next morning on arriving on her floor, I was quickly surrounded by nurses at the main desk. They wanted to know what I did. There was a larger crowd gathering about, to hear my response.

Why, what happened? was my counter question.

She's happy. No more screaming at night. No more complaints of pain.

I thought to myself, all she wanted was hope. And for her, at least, that was the answer.

She passed four days later, still at peace.

Pain is always modulated by the brain.

Did you really do a neurological exam? Damn!

I looked at the resident in a Hospital cross town, that I "covered"

I had been wakened at 2 AM with an urgent call that a lady was in a minor motor vehicle accident. All Imaging studies were normal.

She was awake and conversing, but paralyzed from her neck down.

I drove 35 minutes, in a hurry, to render my opinion. Something was missed!

I stopped before entering her cubicle and turned to the physician who called, and accompanied me to her.

"You say you did a neurological exam, and ascertained nothing. No response to pin prick below the neck, and no voluntary movement of anything?"

He nodded.

I shook my head.

Look, I can see from here she is nicely breathing.

I can also see that she is so large that her arms, extend "beyond" the gurney.

He looked puzzled.

She's holding them by her side, or they would be hanging down (you idiot) !

I entered the cubicle, and introduced myself.

I observed she was responsive, appropriate and moved her eyes about well with no facial paralysis.

I had earlier reviewed the imaging, including that of the Cervical spine before this exam, and was quite comfortable what I was dealing with.

So I worked my magic.

"Look"! I enthusiastically turned to the Resident doctor, "she's starting to move her arms already" (Letting one arm move sideways still held up by the patient)

He remained puzzled, but did not interrupt my performance.

"Dear, it's all coming back very fast now.

Sit up for me (which she did with minimal assistance).

Would you like something to drink?"

She nodded.

"Here, take this cup of water."

She grabbed the glass and began to drink.

Ohhhh, commented the resident.

Slowly, we got her up and walking with guidance, not physical assistance.

"Keep her over night, call me if anything worrisome develops."

I was not happy with his evaluation.

Sometimes hysterical paralysis can be a real bummer.

A physician cannot afford to miss something organic.

So suspicions or not, a bucket list of tests, including Imaging of the most sophisticated nature, blood and urine samples are performed and multiple physician specialties are involved.

And so it was with another patient I saw in consult a few years later.

This man was late middle aged, and stated he had absolutely no function below the waist. He could however have normal bowel movements and there was no urinary incontinence. He had absolutely no feeling below the neck, could easily tolerate a needle in his arm, or deep pain, without apparent perception. There was no history of trauma.

A psychiatrist had cleared the patient of any underlying issues, and another neurologist concluded, he could find nothing to explain this condition.

The patient was quite affable, presenting like a syndrome known as Le Belle Indifference, where there is inappropriate lack of concern for a particular medical condition. While that is seen in a psychiatric disease called a Conversion reaction, I had seen it, at least once before in a patient with frontal brain tumor. Imaging already excluded that possibility.

Psychiatry was adamant this was of organic origin, so the ball was back in our court.

The next day after previously ordered tests were preformed including an EMG and blood and urine results offered no further clues, I had an idea.

By then the patient had been in the hospital more than a week, and frustration about what to do with was obvious with nursing, let alone his referring physician. I sat down next to him, and sympathized with his condition, adding it must be quite stressful for him.   He agreed wholeheartedly.

I then queried, if this situation, even effected his sleep?

He agreed.

Bait taken!

Look, I said. I can't offer any hope that further studies on the "sleep issue" would solve the problem of your paralysis, but would you be interested in having that problem investigated further?

He would agree to all tests that might help solve the riddle.

It was less than 2 hours after that conversation, that once again, the magic worked. I was called by the floor Nursing supervisor who said the patient was standing next to her claiming a "miracle had occurred." And, he was back to normal. He wants to go home.

I told her, she could discharge him in the care of responsible family member, But I wanted to see him back in my office a week later, and to make the appointment before discharge.

What happened?

A sleep study monitors you with video when you are not awake.

People move about, when they are asleep.

The patient immediately understood the consequences of such a study, and elected to avoid any further inquiry.

The following week and a couple months later, repeat neurological exams were normal, and the patient was pleased as peaches.

End of story.

The reader might also be interested in looking up the Hoover sign / Hoover test used to determine if paralysis of one leg is physical or psychiatric. The magic of knowledge works.

Chapter. 14   What's Next?

From his small community came another patient. This one lady was not so lucky. She presented with a brain tumor in the left frontal lobe next to her speech center.
I performed a craniotomy on her while she was "awake", to determine if we were getting too close to that center, in removing the tumor.
It was a semi aggressive type called an Oligodendroglioma.

She did wonderfully. And while she could conceivably have a recurrence, it might take many years. She was ecstatic it was not one of the more malignant types, as were we. There was absolutely no neurological deficit from the tumor, or surgery. Great result.

So when she came back for her two week follow up, I was confused with the irreconcilable tears brought forth by every question.
I stopped and looked closely at her.
"Is something going on I don't know about?"

She paused, then with an even greater abundance of tears, answered,
"They murdered my son!"

I was speechless. How much can a person bear.

I asked further about the case. They knew who killed him, and all the evidence they needed, she was told by the district attorney.

Of course that wouldn't help, except to bring some modicum of closure.

After a lengthy discussion, she left. My mind in a little blizzard going into the next room to evaluate another medical problem.

Kept going back to it the rest of the day. And then some.

Until the following year.

She returned, her affect (facial appearance) appeared flat, emotionless.

I informed her of her follow up MRI which showed absolutely no evidence of recurrence, and noted her pervasive sadness.

I assumed it was still about her son.

So I asked about the case.

She answered,"somehow they lost all the evidence. Nothing will happen".

Again, overwhelming. I was afraid to ask how she was able to go on?

Happily, she did have supportive measures in her local community, though the pain would never leave.

Going from one paragraph to the next, the reader might be experiencing a little bit that a physician, especially a Neurosurgeon, feels going from one room to the next, even one catastrophe to another. Never knowing what the next hour will bring. This is intentional.

From the very highs to the very lows, and back again, ad infinitum.

Or conversely, from the soothing rhythm of such practice to a free fall,

in the blink of an eye.

Not all of the above was chronological, if that was all possible.
But much occurred in that rhythm.

Sometime around then (I don't recall precisely) a gentleman in his mid forties suddenly developed a profound headache, then lost vision in both eyes. On arrival late that night, I saw he not only was bilaterally blind, but had no movement of the right eyeball, and only a little remaining motion in the left. An MRI confirmed Pituitary Apoplexy !
This condition is the result of a brain hemorrhage, inside the pituitary gland, which sits closely against the optic chiasm (nerves to the eyes) and Cavernous sinus (a blood channel where there were nerves to the eye muscles).

By the time, routine evaluation was complete, we had the OR prepped and a transphenoidal hypophysectomy was performed. This surgery uses a approach through the nose to enter a nasal sinus and then the floor of the skull just below the pituitary portion of the brain. Hemorrhage released. Vision restored. Eye muscle function returned in one week. Happiness!

So that's one major reason, why we stay in this field.
Another, I'm sure, is the intellectual and surgical challenges. But we see a lot of interesting lives.

Chapter. 15. No More, Please

Some Neurosurgeons have fought the fight, and dropped out.
My first partner would sometimes disappear after a whole day assisting me on a complex case.   He did this on several occasions, asking me, in late afternoons, if I could handle the rest, without him.
The answer was always, yes. It was helpful to have an assistant, if anything went wrong, or you suddenly had a rare medical problem (like needing a pee break). But not usually critical.
Still, I was curious.

So after a case closed, I called him that night to inquire if he had some routine duties elsewhere, in late afternoons.
He replied he was going to "diesel mechanic school."
Little surprises me anymore.

Indeed upon completion of his training, he divorced, moved to the Beach and became a boat engine mechanic (whatever they're called).

This was not the most bizarre, "retirements" noted.
I can recall a long list of neurosurgeons who changed professions usually at or just after their peak, to play guitar in a coffee house (rumored), become a painter

(good sources confirmed), raise sheep inn Central America (my Professor), and a myriad of other jobs.

All less stress, better life style choices.

More to them.

Chapter. 16.   Still in the Saddle, Must Be Doing Something Right

On this note, a patient arrived with a mild quadriparesis (weakness in all four extremities). A neurosurgeon in one of our large cities noted a damaged Spinal cord and concluded it was an earlier disc herniation in the neck, that still might be dynamically significant, and related to his condition.
So he did an anterior cervical fusion. This is an operation through the front of the neck going between the carotid artery artery and jugular vein on one side, and the Esophagus (swallowing pipe) windpipe on the other, to enter the disc, remove it (now almost always with a microscope) and fuse the joint after decompression.

He was wrong.

The area of spinal cord injury had some mass effect (our first clue) that a small disc herniation was not the cause of his neurological deterioration,
or Imaging abnormality.

He was on cortisone for continued gradual deterioration, and an extensive medical evaluation failed to reveal the source of this problem.
I concluded it could be a growth, or tumor.

Surgery was performed entering the spine from behind and removing the smallest portion of abnormal tissue from the spinal cord, for pathology to exam.

It turned out he had Sarcoidosis (where have you heard this before?)

There was no specific treatment for this condition, and he was left on

his steroids for now, with follow up locally.

A few months later I received a phone call from an Attorney in a large

Southern city.   He asked if I would speak to him about this case.

I initially hesitated, but then agreed on a limited basis.

To summarize.

He first asked if I was the operating surgeon, and replied yes.

Then he asked if the local neurosurgeon operated on the wrong problem,

I was forced to agree.

Finally he asked me if any permanent harm occurred because of that

Neurosurgeons actions.

I replied, NO.

So much for any lawsuit.

Wait a minute.

Then he asked, if I knew who he was?

I answered, I didn't know his firm, and would he repeat his name?

It was familiar.

He went on to say, he was a Neurosurgeon in another part of my state,

who became a plaintiff attorney.

Wow!

I remembered him then, and understood his transformation.

But still, thought. Wow!

I guess, If you can't beat them, join them.

Isn't all this interesting? I thought it was, so I decided to write this book. Amazing that it is, I'm sure all Neurosurgeons have equally fascinating stories, maybe little time to tell them, or energy.

Thing is, I believe it gets harder as the surgeon matures in dealing with some of the more horrendous cases. I suspect that is the opposite for some folks, and my comment implies no disrespect. By "harder", I mean you increasingly identify with the patient and family, so horrendous news as to a prognosis, colors your weeks to follow (sometimes much longer). Maybe, you just identify more with the victim.

A few years after I started my practice, a 17 year old came to the Emergency room, following a severe motorcycle wreck. Helmet was crushed, as was his skull. But he had a large shift of brain to the right from immense brain swelling on the left and some areas of hemorrhage. He had blown a pupil on the left suggesting he was herniating his brain and would not survive much longer. His breathing was irregular. Medication to control the shift of brain and hyperventilation failed to slow the rapid progression.

I sat down with his folks. They were torn asunder, explaining he left home a few weeks earlier, after an argument (possibly about money). They would do anything to save their son now, and implored me to do so as well.

I offered a decompression craniotomy with distant hope of survival, but even if that happened it would not guarantee a reasonably functioning person. Still, they urged me, to do what I could. "Money was no problem".

They did come from a very wealthy suburb, and understood the offer, though it would and could not, change my approach.
I went to surgery that night, hoping for the best. It was not to happen.

On opening the skin, brain squirted out, and continued to do so, down the drapes, into a bucket. The patient of course had skull fractures, but also the canvas like dura surrounding the brain was torn, and the brain pulverized. This was in a large portion of the left frontal area, and meant he would be devastated neurologically under the most optimum of circumstances. I decompressed what I could, leaving skull portions out and a generous patch over the torn membrane.

Maybe the reader might be inclined to think loss of brain matter to a Neurosurgeon is accepted as part of the job.   Just the opposite !
If anything, this holy land, is even more sacred to those who must pass by it, or through it, to cure.

I was comforted, yes, comforted, when he did not survive a few more hours. Of course his folks were devastated.
He was their "everything".
Or was he?

My office had sent a bill to his home and the parents replied he was a minor and they had no responsibility for paying it.

They were correct of course. Still, maybe? I was even more sympathetic to this young lad.

It brought me back to my Navy days, when a sign hung as you entered the Neurosurgery ward "Get your son a motorcycle for his last birthday".

Swinging now to a more cheerful event (this is very much like a neurosurgeon's practice with extreme highs and extreme lows).

Sometimes the elderly are the most fun. Unless they are in failing cognitive health, decisions at times, are easier in regards to major surgery.

I was seeing a lady about age 90 for spinal stenosis (narrowing of the spine crushing the spinal cord) in this case, from arthritis.

She was noted to be Quadriparetic (remember, weakness in all four extremities) and had problems walking, even with assistance..

Because of her age and comorbidities, I placed her in a cervical collar and followed her with repetitive neurological examinations.

She went downhill fast.

Within the month she no longer could feed herself, care for herself, or walk with assistance. She started having problems breathing.

Her primary care physician admitted her and consulted me, and, for a second opinion, another neurosurgical group.

The other consultant wrote, her age, medical condition and severity of neurological complaints would prohibit any successful decompression.

He commented, surgery was "not recommended."

I sat down with the patient.

She well understood the risks involved, especially death from a myriad of causes with the surgical option. I asked her to choose.
Did she want to stay this way, or bluntly put, go for it?
Without hesitation she answered. This is no life, I'd rather die.

I took her to surgery and performed a successful decompression of the cervical spine. Before discharge a few days later, she was feeding herself, and could ambulate "without" assistance.

We won that time. But, it could have gone wrong.
Either way, it's what I would have chosen for myself, under those conditions.

When young, many of us crave excitement and adventure.
As we age sometimes these can be the euphemisms for terror.
So then gracefully we search for, control and predictability.
An illusion, but worth one's efforts.

Most of our surgeries, even large ones, fall into that last category.
They do become routine. Outcomes predictable. This is what enables a senior neurosurgeon to make wise decisions, that might allude the less experienced, though gifted, junior colleagues.
They in turn have the advantage of stamina, and new thought.
Together, they can be awesome.

I can only imagine Neurosurgery 50 or 100 years from now.

Actually nobody, probably can accurately predict its course.

When I just started out in the 1970s, Lasers where very fashionable.

Despite this, it was seldom used in the last thirty years, because

other options were deemed more satisfactory.

Different specialties would have different experiences with various

advancements, some found them useful, others not.

I think the most significant advance (and there have been many) for

for my specialty, has been "Imaging, with localization for the brain and spine".

First CAT scans, then MRIs and even much more coming on-line at the present,

enable the surgeon to diagnose and localize the problem, with smaller

(minimally invasive surgeries) dominating.

Interesting, that I used minimally invasive operations in the late 1970s.

But they are more accurate, and successful, now.

At the end of may surgical career for instance, I was doing one or two level lumbar

fusions with instrumentation's, as "out patient". I reflect on the days when a

simple Laminectomy kept patients in the hospital 5 days or more (even in the 1980s).

Of course just because we can, so to speak, build a ship in a bottle, doesn't

mean it's the best option, to do it that way.   Hopefully that analogy is

understood, when we are talking about surgeries. It's the end results, that count.

We all expected in the 1950s, that by the year 2000 we would have "flying cars."

That didn't occur, but the internet and smart phones did. I would vote for them

over the flying contraceptions, any day.

So science does not follow a direct line. And much of we have today, even in our sophisticated medical society is pure rubbish. I won't go into that discussion here, That might get too emotional. But the vulnerable are preyed upon, just as they had been in the nineteenth century, when the charlatans of the day offered magical cures (more than a few of these are still around).

Today, we have a new generation of physicians. Some are simply awesome. They are brilliant and hard workers. I believe most Neurosurgeons fall into that category.

However, I have noticed a shift for the many young physicians, in other Medical specialties. Their argument is "I'm not interested in money, just a good life style". This translated, means, I want a 9 to 5 job.

With the consolidation of Medicine today, large hospitals own many Physicians' practices, and less and less physicians own, their own.
This employment arrangement, creates such opportunity for a no call schedule, or limited one. It is especially advantageous for women Physicians, who also wish to raise a family. They are paradigm shifts, nevertheless. Some, like telemedicine, I expect will become even more prevalent, now that we have had the Covid 19 crisis. Extended Medical assistants, like Physician assistants, and Nurse practitioners, I think will be a very positive step in balancing the work situation for many in mine, and other specialties.

Certain patients will like the changes, others will not. Recent patient physician relationships have changed at a historically dramatic speed. I suspect, in the immediate future, such changes will be more widespread and even more dramatic. The world will see a different physician entirely in 50 years.

Surgeons will operate on patients thousands of miles away, by robotics,

And AI will make many of the medical decisions our family doctor presently offers.

And that, will be routine. It's not flying cars, but I suppose that will come eventually.

We will continue to refine what is meant by "peer review, and evidence based" studies. Medical legal laws will change with technological shifts.

Medical rationing will be a certainty (hopefully minimized to extreme circumstances, as it is today).

Hang on! It's going to be quite a ride.

But, hopefully not back to the days of Charity hospitals.

Chapter. 17.   CONTRADICTIONS

(Some views on my specialty)

In this time of minimally invasive this and that, a surprising trend has occurred. The "opposite".

Neurosurgeons probably have the most challenging training (Residency) of any physicians specializing. They are young, athletic and bright, and maybe most important of all, driven.
They usually want to do the most difficult procedures and complex tasks. Their seven or so years after medical school, has made them a different person.

One could argue, that their own preexisting personality found this path, but the path nevertheless, will change them, their families, and acquaintances. Most residents I suspect, are not from the city area, let alone the city, where they do their training . Friendships cannot be maintained frequently, because they are away working, and the relations not nourished. Babies are born and may have little time with the parent, because of hours spent in the hospital. Family members pass, funerals and weddings are missed. Things change.

Even upon completion of the program, the new Neurosurgeon may choose a different state to practice, from whence he came.

"You can't go back home."
        And you can't go back to who you were.

One can't undo these years away, physically, emotionally, and return.
Their world has changed. They are different.
Not blinking, a recent neurosurgical graduate returned to his program to give a talk about his practice, after one year. I was there, listening to what happened, more aware than he, of what transformed.

He explained, "yesterday I saw 56 patients, then did two emergency Craniotomies though the night, caught a little nap, and drove six hours to give this talk, putting this presentation together (with slides) 2 hours ago."

He said smiling, that his wife has on the calendar the couple times he is home for dinner each month.
Yet here I sat, wishing it was me, again.

Young, so full of energy, performing impossible tasks routinely.
Handsome, well spoken and in control, my, my.
He certainly does have the candy store.

What is his destiny?
We certainly need people like that, want and admire them.
But can he "hold it together", for a year, years, decades, like I have?

Wouldn't put it past him. But wouldn't bet on it, either.

Somewhere in time, we reflect.
I have been with my lady 60 years. I think this is perhaps unusual for this field. Relationships need replenishment constantly. Are they capable, or so inclined?
Not a measure of human success, I suppose.
And how does one measure happiness?
Pride in accomplishments (well deserved by the majority) really is not happiness, at least not in my book.

But the accomplishments are real, and maybe that which alone keeps some going (I can name names). Some really can't survive in society outside the operating room, others look for new spouses to "find the dream". Some work until they no longer can.

A vendor told me about a neurosurgeon in another state, operating well into his seventies. Eventually one day after a particularly long case, he collapsed on the floor of the operating room, exhausted. "I'm Done. What am I going to do now?" He asked no one.

It seems to me an inordinate amount of surgeons pass away a few months, after they retire. In these cases, I saw them all go "cold turkey".

The first question I asked another Neurosurgeon on my entering private practice was "what is retirement?" He just joined that club.
He told me he planned to travel, read a lot and do things he couldn't,

because of his previously hectic schedule. Unfortunately, that was not to be, the following month passing from an unsuspected brainstem Glioma (Malignant brain tumor in a very nasty spot).

Tomorrow, truly is not promised.
But they must "live the day".

Meanwhile, despite the above tangent, such talented creatures demand the finest in surgical tools, offer the finest in surgical skills, relish the biggest most complicated cases.
Which brings me to my number one "pet peeve."

The OVERUSE of spinal "fusion" surgery.

In this discussion, it should be recognized that fusion surgery, under the proper indications, can be life changing (in a good way).
I would also like to state up front, that it is a well accepted operation in the neurosurgical community and, this was a good part of my practice.

But let's start with, what I believe to be the commonest operation on the neck for a cervical disc herniation, causing pain down the neck into the arm, sometimes to the fingers, not rarely with a mild degree at least, of paralysis. The patient frequently wakes up one morning finding he or she has a "crick" in the neck. It won't go away, and soon the pain is quite bad.

Conservative treatment is usually indicated initially, with such drugs as cortisone, or anti-inflammatory medication. Some physicians might add analgesics (pain meds) and muscle relaxants. If it doesn't go away, and an MRI scan confirms a herniated disc or arthritis/spur pressing on the appropriate nerve, surgery might then be considered, especially if weakness is noted in the muscle, supplied by the crushed nerve. It can be either from the front of the neck (anterior) or from behind the neck (posterior). Both have been shown to be equally effective.

The posterior approach, usually does not need concomitant fusion, although I see an ominous trend to do that as well. The anterior does.
Both are reasonably safe operations, the majority of times.
Yet, I believe most surgeons in my experience, highly prefer the anterior route.

What's the pros and cons?
First we will mention, only to set aside, throughout my career, insurance carriers have paid the surgeon about twice as much to do the anterior approach, than the posterior. It's important to stop here, and emphasize that sometimes, this is the ONLY option. For instance if there is spinal cord compression from a "central" disc, it is not safe to try removing this from a posterior approach.

But the "majority" of disc herniations or spurs causing pain and/or paralysis in an upper extremity are on the side, easily recompressed from behind "without" fusion.

In addition, multiple levels can be decompressed from the posterior approach without doing a single fusion, through one incision! So why is the frontal approach usually the first thought for your surgeon? I suspect there are several reasons for this, in no particular order.

Let's consider the "posterior approach" with the patient in the "sitting position" and the surgeon operating from behind.

First of all, a surgeon with short arms, would have considerable limitations performing the posterior operation using a microscope, as now would be the routine. The operating microscope takes room. The surgeons arms need to go around the scope. If the patient was prone (down on their chest) the scope Is bent. However, if the patient is sitting it is straight…making the patient a few inches further, longer arms an advantage. Simple as that.

Even the added comfort of an arm rest (usually the back of the operating table) occupies space.

Furthermore, positioning of the patient, and (used by some anesthesiologists when the operation is done with the patient "sitting") a Central line, for IV etc., takes time.

Also, there is the unreasonable fear of air being sucked into an open blood vessel (air emboli). I can assure the reader that I have done this operation routinely and frequently (more than anyone in my state) without ever having a significant event of that sort…..over 35 years !
So why is there this fear?

Because such complications "can occur" when operating "on the brain" with the patient sitting. (I suspect not uncommonly, if near rigid venous structures). Even then, with appropriate precautions, this can be made safer.

So why not operate with the patient prone (on their tummy) for the "posterior" approach?

Well, then the neck has to be flexed, (chin down) so the initial incision is well below the level of disc herniation, the cut often extending into the upper thoracic spine. Think of it this way. The neck is bent somewhat on the chest while the patient lies on his stomach. Problems?

Well, first of all, the head of the operating table has to be removed, the patient fixed in a clamp, AND THEN (here's the important part) the operating table needs to be elevated at the "head of the bed", with feet end down, or the surgeon would have his own neck kinked sideways, the same amount as the patient's neck is flexed. Uncomfortable.

Placing the head in a clamp, positioning of the patient sitting, and a central venous line, probably takes more than 20 minutes, total. Considering the surgery itself, may be one hour each, you see the temptation to go from the front of the neck, especially if the surgeon has many operations to do that day. After all, the pain relief should be the same. So why worry?

My gosh, this is an answer searching for a question !
Yep, surgeons can now use a device to avoid fusion when going from the front of the neck. They can replace the disc removed, with an "Artificial Disc," instead of fusing. A much more complicated, more expensive operation, with its own set of risks, including the device at times, unfortunately fusing the spine, anyways.. Some believe fusion can cause problems with early deterioration of the disc below, and especially the disc above.

But for the vast majority of people, I would not be too concerned about that for a one level fusion, even two levels (though the behind approach, seems more physiological, and less invasive).

Now we got some speed. Consider that a good number of patients may eventually have a three levels fusion! There are six levels in the neck (seven vertebra) spine, and the top line has little to do with flexion and extension, performing rotation of the neck. In the case of a three level fusion "half your neck is fused"! Is that bad?

There is a legitimate diagnosis called "post fusion syndrome", as your insurance company and Medicare, are well aware. The more levels fused, the more likely you are, to develop this problem.

The symptoms are unremitting back of the neck pain (for neck fusion) sometimes spreading into the proximal muscles known as the trapezius, and even into the upper thoracic spine. What causes this?

Patients having fusion of the spine, seldom notice any major decreased range of motion. That's because "other" spine levels (discs) compensate by over-extending their physiologically designed rage of motion.

Much like extending your elbow backwards, on a block of wood with palm up.
You CAN do so, if someone sat on your wrist for several months.
The joint is not meant for that, of course, and the result would be elbow pain.

A few years ago, a national newspaper (pretty sure it was the Wall Street Journal) discussed a pending study to determine which would be the best approach for Cervical discs herniations. The anterior approach was mentioned with fusion, and an artificial disc for the neck, and finally, a posterior FUSION.

They didn't even mention, a behind the neck simple operation (without fusion) proven as effective with less risks, I would argue, than the other type surgeries.

I once heard a talk about how we must consider going from behind the spine, or surgeons will "forget" how to do them. Of course, they wouldn't forget. It just wouldn't be on their radar, as a viable option. We are enamored with technology, and to some extent, if it's not more complex, how can it be better?

In addition, a good operation now is being ruined (my word) with physicians that find they can successfully fuse multiple levels from behind without much additional risk (except for post fusion syndrome, which I presently see in abundance).

Getting back to dollars. I estimate I had a seven figure loss over the years, for performing posterior approach surgeries, which I believed better for the patient in the long run, in most cases. A little extra time in the OR, considerably less renumeration, but often worth it, If you're the patient.

There is an analogous situation in fusing the lumbar spine (low back).
The two main reasons given for such surgery, are an unstable spine, as in one with subluxation (spondylolisthesis) or, a surgeon believes decompressive surgery, say for a spur, would take enough boney or ligamentous structure away that surgery may make you unstable.
Trauma, and tumors are less common indications.

My issue with that scenario, is that some surgeons believe they cannot decompress the openings, where the nerves come out sideways, called neuroforamen without causing instability.

Since I have done this for almost forty years, with seldom such an issue, I worry that this is too aggressive. At risk of becoming too technical, let us just say, that I conclude fusion of the spine surgery is overdone.

Opposing opinions accepted.

Being in private practice, until recently, was not the platform to address such issues. But one certainly is exposed to trends by way of continued education, whether by print, internet, or meetings. I just don't agree with the reasons given for so many fusions, which seem unnecessarily aggressive.

Always ask for alternatives, and a second opinion. Especially, if the word "fusion" is mentioned.

So much for the lecture. Thanks for allowing me to "vent."

Chapter. 18.   We Thought Problems Solved

Heart stopping…not the patient's, the surgeons! He must remain cool in extremely adverse situations in the operating room. Maybe like a pilot who flew his entire career without incidenct, then one day has a flame-out of both engines.

More likely, by far however, would be like a bomber mission over Germany in WWII. You have advanced warning there will be trouble, which gives you time to prepare, but it doesn't lessen the stress.

I've had my share. So has every neurosurgeon.

One I recall quite vividly, was a patient who had a brain hemorrhage from a basilar tip aneurysm. This is a bulb like expansion on the artery like a weak part in an old ballon tire, in this case already starting to leak.

Nowadays, such an event would possibly be handled differently, but thirty something years ago, surgery was the only real option available, besides hoping for the best with supportive care.

The operation proceeded as planned, quite smoothly, the beast dissected clearly despite a very small opening/access for a clip to occlude it.

This aneurysm was located below the center of the brain, a very hard to get to location.

The moment of truth arrived, and the clip was applied.

That's normally the time a surgeon breathes a sigh of relief.

In this case however, I had considerable trouble detaching the aneurysm clip holder. Perhaps the clip rotated somewhat along the vessel, and there was little room to expand the holder, never knew for certain, why I had this difficulty. But, I became desperate, fast. I was afraid the clip holder would twist with my maneuvers to remove it, and tear off the tip of the aneurysm. All would be over, in a very fast, bloody explosion.

After a few prayers, and gentle manipulation, I finally could deliver the holder from its position. Patient survived.

Sometimes, you do expect the worst, (one ALWAYS has to be prepared for that) and nothing bad happens. Or, it happens much later.

Decades back when stereotactic radiosurgery (focused radiation) was in its infancy, a young woman appeared in the ER with a small brain hemorrhage, An arteriogram was done (this was before MRIs and MRAs were available). I couldn't believe my eyes. Most of right side of the brain was occupied by a large Arteriovenous Malformation. I would never touch that!

Having said this, the actual problem was much smaller. The nidus of this, or precise area between the high pressure arterial supply and low pressure, but extremely engorged venous supply, was the culprit. We could never clearly determine with 100% accuracy the shape and exact location, but had a good idea.

She was neurologically intact, and stable.

After a period of observation I discharged her and made plans of a special type of radiation to clot off the large malformation, in another state.

Problem was, taming that monster, could take a year... if successful.
In the meantime a fatal recurrent hemorrhage could occur.
We were fortunate, to a degree.

She tolerated the treatment nicely and follow up exams with a CAT scan, found no recurrent hemorrhage, when checked periodically.
Then about 18 months later, she suffered another hemorrhage in association with a seizure. Repeat Arteriogram was depressing. Most of the huge blood vessel malformation was unchanged. I had further discussion with other neurosurgeons, and a repeat radiation course was the consensus. Once more she remained neurologically intact, despite the seizures, and now intermittently severe headaches.

Still another year passed. Now with the perspective of a new imaging machine called MRI, we could see her abnormality in a different manner. The malformation still appeared present, though not high flow, and a further problem was found. Her brain was immensely swollen on the right side with some shift of that hemisphere to the left. Surprisingly, she remained neurologically normal.

We tried some courses of Decadron (a steroid) hoping to lessen the swelling, without any improvement seen on initial follow up. After much soul searching, our plan was to sit back and pray that eventually the swelling would lessen.

I continued to follow her for another year or more, with what I thought
was indeed, slight lessening, of brain swelling.
Then she was lost to follow up…until a few years later.

Now in her mid twenties, she arrived one night to our ER, comatose.
A week or so earlier, she delivered a baby, which went uneventfully, but
in the previous twenty-four hours had gone progressively downhill.
Her right pupil was "blown" or dilated, suggesting brain herniation, and
She had lost some of her cranial nerve function, on that side. The brain swelling
and shift, was far worse. I had to do something.

This was a most unpleasant decision. An arteriogram suggested a
good deal of the AVM (blood vessel malformation) was now occluded,
and brain swelling was thought likely related to her two previous treatments
of radiation to that side of the brain.

The multiple vessels again, were the size of a grown man's index finger.
and their nest, that of a woman's fist.
What if they were only partially occluded? Would taking the remaining
malformation cause further swelling of the brain?
Turns out this monster was so large, that at the time of craniotomy,
removing it and a non significant tip of the temporal lobe was all
that was necessary.

Didn't know that when, opening the skull and dura (membrane beneath the skull).
it looked formidable. No obvious pulsations, and a fine needle placed inside

one of the large vessels (followed by bigger needles) failed to find any evidence this monster, still lived.

Nevertheless, sphincters were once again tight, when I cut across them with a scalpel. So much volume of aberrant blood vessels (now rock hard and devoid of blood) was removed, that a vast cavity was made, and this is how the brain swelling issue resolved.

The patient awoke, recovering fully, and after a few years follow up with Imaging, showed no residual AVM, discharged.

No doubt many neurosurgeons have had equal or more "eventful" times. But a final case should be mentioned, that somehow to me, seems similar. Well, the part that was similar was that I had another young lady about age 20 with another rare aneurysm, this time in the posterior fossa (back portion of the brain).

A search of literature could find only four such patients reported, who were operated on, and these were all in Europe.
Being in private practice, but holding privileges at a University hospital, as well as my own institution, I decided to perform the surgery there.

Admittedly, this was done with the purpose of having additional minds, so in case the worst happened, there was a sound legal defense.

I assure the reader what follows happened exactly, as described.

Following long discussions with the patient and family, and the University physician who would be assisting me during the surgery, we soon thereafter, brought her to the hospital for the planned procedure.

As usual, Neurosurgical residents in training, would perform the opening of the head /skull. Then, I would perform the actual procedure. This was quite routine, and she came to the operating theater, and was put to sleep uneventfully.

After I was confident the patient was positioned properly, I received a message from the Neurosurgical chief of the University, asking if I could come to his office. I agreed, noting that the neurosurgical residents now were beginning the operation. Entering the skull and obtaining some exposure, would take awhile, so I felt comfortable with them performing the lesser part of the procedure, and went up to his office.

The Chief wasted no time in informing me the I would NOT perform this surgery.

What?

Are you. Crazy? (Didn't use that term).
The patient understands I'm the surgeon, the operative permit was signed with my name as surgeon, this is absurd.
Now, not only the stress of performing a rare brain surgery on a young lady, but now this ridiculous issue being thrown at me, while the patient was asleep, and her brain being exposed.
Next to me sat the "prior" Chief of Neurosurgery for that institution.
I looked his way, but no clue as his thoughts.

"He will be the surgeon". the present chief said, nodding to former.

Explain! I demanded. (Probably in less polite terms).

The present chief replied, well doctor, our neurosurgeons are "self insured," And you have a malpractice carrier, that wouldn't cover an event in this Hospital".

I was numb.

The silence not reflecting my thoughts.

"You just found that out now"? I screamed.

There was no answer. Guess it didn't matter.

By then I wasn't a happy camper.

This is unethical, I yelled. There is no excuse.

"Call them up now"! I demanded. Whoever your carrier is, the patient is asleep and being operated on, as we speak.

I sensed a long winded response as to why that couldn't be done.

The Chief simply replied, "I'm sorry, that's the way it is."

No! I retaliated, now extremely angry.

There's a patient in the middle of surgery, and you have no leverage here.

There was a pause, probably seconds, but it felt like hours.

The "former" Chief spoke up.

"What if", he began. then stopped.

I can't tell you how much I hung on the words to follow.

"What if, I assisted him as planned, and took personal responsibility for any actions during the surgery"?

This man's my hero !

I looked back to present Chief. Agreed, I asked?

Well, if he wishes to be responsible…

Didn't hear the final few words, I already was out of there back to the OR.

Within the hour the other Neurosurgeon (my Hero) joined the team.

Words could not describe how much I appreciated this gesture.

This was a Neurosurgeon !

That's how we act!

How can you thank such a man?

The patient did well.

That's how!

Chapter. 19.   Being "That" Neurosurgeon

These patient snippets, are not the only fascinating stories I recall, over the last 50 years. (Still have some real doozies).
Indeed, every patient had his or her own story to tell, of the tens of thousands I have seen in my lifetime.

They may not all have been as interesting as the above, though some really could have been included in the list.
But each of us will almost certainly be a patient at some time, in our lives.
I'm sure we all would like to think that moment was important not only for us, but the physician as well.

When I contemplate a lifetime as a physician, as opposed to another career, it concludes with one thought. I have seen the best in people, I strongly suspect other occupations less so. Attorneys, for instance, probably see the worst in us, and other occupations, in between.

I'm convinced, we all have a good side, and a nefarious one, in varying proportions. And this layer cake varies throughout our life. Humans are complex creatures, who continually have surprised me, with their resilience, unselfishness, bravery, and understanding.

It could be said, there are patients who you know are trouble.

They are usually easy to spot. Someone who has been in five car accidents, with a lawsuit against the other driver for each incident. Likewise, someone that is very hostile to your staff, could be equally so, to the physician.

Of course, having said that, I can readily understand why some patients are frustrated, even angry, with the medical establishment. Rarely, they might indeed have been mistreated, more commonly, misdiagnosed. At times, no matter who you are, you're in the bullseye. One just has to understand that this is part of being a care provider.

I can recall one patient who screamed at me, his pain was so intolerable. He promised if I didn't fix him, he would commit suicide. Fortunately, I was able to ascertain his problem and present a solution.

Not so fast.

The insurance company refused to certify his planned surgery, explaining on the phone when I appealed their decision, that he was suicidal and this is why he couldn't deal with his pain. He was depressed.

That may have been another time I exploded a bit, speaking to the insurance clone, who was quoting from their Bible of guidelines (that was made by physicians like me).

This is not in your cookbook, I explained. He has that severe of pain! I have the tests that show what is causing his agony.

They relinquished.

Surgery performed.

Big bear hug, from the patient afterwards.

My specialty rules!

This week, "as I am writing this narrative", two more related incidents occurred ! (They continue coming.)

Frustrations from patients in pain, or paralysis, or for almost any serious complaint, are common and understandable.

The first was a middle aged lady who had some back, but mainly hip and groin pain, for fifteen years. She had seen many physicians, even receiving "spinal blocks" that didn't help. She was at her wits end. Doing Telemedicine, and asking her to perform a Patrick test, crossing her legs a certain way, it was obvious with all spinal Imaging being negative, that this pain was coming from her hips. This was never evaluated by any of her many previous physicians, including a "pain specialist".

MRI scan of her hips shows "avascular necrosis", as the source of unrelenting pain. We had the answer immediately!

She was happy but…why in God's name, wasn't this found by her previous Doctors, all those years?

Am I going to be an expert witness in some lawsuit? We'll see. I did explain that In some instances, similar symptoms can occur from both conditions.

Hope that helped lessen her frustration.

Even more exasperating, was a woman with stage IV Metastatic breast

Cancer. The recurrence was just found a day before, and you can imagine

the anguish she was presently enduring. More than that. She had extreme pain

in an arm, not controlled by even heavy narcotics.

The Cervical spine was said to be the source by the referring specialist.

It wasn't   Her pain was coming from the brachial plexus, a network of

Nerves in the chest behind the clavicle. The Cervical MRI was not impressive.

While her case, somewhat more complex than will be discussed, noted

a pleural effusion (a good deal of fluid on her lung, from the cancer), I hoped

that drainage already planned by her Oncologist, would lessen the discomfort.

It didn't.

She, I believe, was certain my diagnose was in error !

While I myself was confident we understood the problem, it was necessary to

convince her other specialists, and even the patient.   A brachial plexus MRI was

done which confirmed my diagnosis. The Plexus was swollen and inflamed!

She questioned why a local MRI of the chest missed the diagnosis, and

I explained certain "sequences", or if you will, Apps, driving the machine,

were necessary to visualize such an unusual problem.

I felt good, she had an answer. Her specialists couldn't deny the

diagnosis any longer. And while, the prognosis was well understood by

this intelligent lady, we now had certainty, to explain her pain.

Sometimes, we don't know, what we don't know.

But sometimes we simply don't agree, with what our physician is saying,

Now that is frustrating! So she is relieved somewhat, in ascertaining the cause for her condition. Less frustration, and a "plan" during this most trying of times. That's what she sought. Onward.

Her Oncologist can feel more comfortable as well, in addressing this issue. An Image, is worth a thousand words. It was apparently, necessary here.

Other patients just need kid gloves. Like the one that starts out saying they understand I am the world's best for their problem, after seeing dozens of other physicians for their complaint. And they know I will find the cause for their symptoms.

It really is cool, when you are "that" physician who finds the missing clue, and can diagnosis and treat their years long quest. (See two examples back).

I'd like to think that was my strength. But there are many great physicians out there, so this becomes less likely, after the first few seen. Expectations dashed, are frustrating for patient and physician alike.

I'm not sure what empathy is. If it is the understanding that this individual who seeks your help desperately needs you, then how could we not have that emotion. If it is the comprehension of what they are going through, this is essential for any physician. If it is the recognition that they are like you, and deserve respect, of course. If you have any humanity, what other choice do you have? And sometimes empathy can be difficult.

For instance, when you have you to do what is best for the patient, including accepting them as a patient in the first place, knowing a lawsuit will accompany your best efforts. This happens.

Even when "not" the target, physicians try to avoid these Legal situations. They're seldom a pleasant task.

These experiences have changed me and my practice. For clarification, when I first began my career, I believed what was needed most for my patients, was an accurate diagnosis and perfect surgical technique.
Towards the last half of my surgical life, I focused more strongly, on what patients "really wanted".
There is a fine, but HUGE line, between the above two goals.

Let me explain. It means considering the entire patient. Not just the diagnosis, but their age, medical condition, and most of all, needs.

A simple example would be a man who has metastatic Prostate cancer, with perhaps a few years survival time. We'll use that diagnosis to illustrate our point.

If he has a spine problem causing pain, a small surgery that eliminates the pain for those years, would be preferred to a large intervention, that would give relief for decades. The larger one not eliminated, because he couldn't tolerate it. It just wasn't necessary.

Picking the best option for the patient obviously requires knowledge of the patient beyond their medical history.
A patient who is 20 years old may find surgery which would allow him to run, essential. But for an 80 year old, running, may not be high on the list of activities in which they wish to participate. And surgery, with its risks, expense, and recovery time, not necessary at all. This is a real example and may be found when a patient

has weakness of a gastrocnemius muscle of spinal origin. If in no pain, an elderly person may choose just to walk, rather than than "fixing the problem".

The number of examples for such consideration would by themselves fill a book, and not without controversy. But, the best guide is the "Patient decides". Yes, there are caveats, but that's where we start.

Chapter. 20.   A Farewell.

I think it appropriate to consider the families, who sometimes are forced to endure even more than the patient themselves.

A patient with a malignant brain tumor surely suffers immensely. Generally however, there is little discomfort, just gradual progression of paralysis and the knowledge that the end is near.

The families however witness the deterioration, and watch them slowly slip into coma. During this deterioration, there is usually need for further assistance, with the need for a wheelchair, help in transferring to a bed or chair, diapers, bathing, economic stress, and watching a loved one disappear.

Arguably they suffer as much, especially if the victim has a family with children. The little ones have to be talked to, and witness the horrors of the prognosis. How is this handled? It varies, but, rest assured, this is a very unpleasant time, usually months, sometimes a year or more. And these children if young, don't fully understand what is happening. If older, it could be even more an emotional dagger.

Another example is sometimes found accompanying Alzheimer's Disease.
The family may be under more stress than the patient.
And so forth.

Suddenly we find heroes, that don't deserve or want the challenge.
It is forced upon them. Their world changes, as caregivers.

We could go on and on, such as certain neurological congenital deformities where the family strives to care for an infant that remains much like one, until his forties when the parents can no longer help, or aren't there.

Our society now is more supportive of these individuals, than when I first began my journey. But It remains a terribly difficult journey.
I cannot tell you how satisfying it is, for us to lessen this burden.
Better yet, to have an answer.

A final patient vignette is in order here. On presentation, a family was desperate for assistance, I doubt expecting any real help. We, on the other hand were optimistic we could, but the "cure" found us confronted by a patient who had his own tale.

Some years back, I seen in my clinic, a gentleman accompanied by several family members. He was in a wheelchair, unable to walk, incontinent of urine, and demented to the point of being unable to speak, save for a few garbled words.

The deterioration began slowly at first, but hastened in the last few months.
His occupation had been an engineer, requiring significant daily mental challenges, which prior to this illness, all agreed, were performed impeccably.

The diagnosis was suspect, in the first few minutes of my exam, and confirmed later that week by a brain MRI. He had NPH.

Remember a case presented earlier, with Normal Pressure Hydrocephalus? Well, in my practice, I have seen many, and indeed it's a real joy to find, not only the cause for any dementia, but to have a viable treatment option.

For this diagnosis, you recall, a shunt is placed in the hollow cavities of the brain named "ventricles", usually draining the spinal fluid into the abdominal cavity by a long subcutaneous catheter. It is one of the easiest neurosurgical operations to perform, learned early, by mosts residents training to become neurosurgeons.

Weeks after he had this "shunt surgery" the patient returned. The results were spectacular! He not only could walk without assistance, he could hop and jump, with great agility. All incontinence resolved, and his language skills were back to normal. We were overjoyed, as was the patient and his entire family. (Indeed, many referrals came from this individual, afterwards.)

I could be forgiven the opportunity to relish in such a success, spending extra time with him, learning of his vast accomplishments, since the procedure. But what he mentioned at the end of our conversation, was indelibly remembered. He said, and I quote to the best of my recollection. "I knew I could not think." How is that possible? In the throughs of his mental decline, there was recognition of his cognitive limitations. Amazing ! A patient who has a severe problem thinking, could "think" about his problem, even when he could not longer speak.

There is much to learn about brain function. I doubt we have even scratched the surface of understanding that organ. Periodically, I reflect back on his statement, and ponder, the "how?"

The study of the brain and spine is the most challenging quest I can imagine. Early on, we can be lost in the extreme (read that amazing) complexity and wonders of our chosen field. Witness the above case.

And for most most of us, I believe the physical and emotional, let alone intellectual prerequisites, initially form a protective barrier from the reality of our Specialty. But, such an insular cone, usually only delays a short time, before realization of harsh realty. Our patients are like us. They are us.
As we mature in this field, I suggest, for many, if not most, this barrier is breached quite rapidly.

I have witnessed however, that some of us still can remain above "identifying" with their patients. For those surgeons, it may be advantageous, as long as perfection rules their character. You don't want to worry about destroying a patient with the slip of a hand. Admittedly repetitive surgeries can serve the function like a shy performer, who after his first hundred appearances before a large audience, becomes comfortable on stage.

The problem then, is one of perfection and character of the surgeon.
If he accepts less than his best (good enough for government work) the patient can suffer terribly. A very busy surgeon might be more vulnerable. Remember however, a surgeon who performs a surgical technique often generally should have better results, than when he does such cases rarely.

And there is the gifted neurosurgeon who discusses with great pride, the risks he takes performing a certain elective surgery, because he has the Cahonas. Again, I could name names.

What the hell?   What is he thinking?

There are safer alternatives! You may not get your name in the news,

But really, that's not the point.

A fast surgeon. A surgeons speed in performing an operation improves over time, like practicing a piano, or skiing.

But to relish speed over accuracy, and thoroughness, diminishes the results. It may impress the nurses in the OR……again, not the point.

The trendy surgeon. Yes, even in our field there are fleeting "wonder surgeries" (or not so fleeting). I have seen many a novel technique on the spine last fashionably for a few, even a dozen or more years, then disappear.

What happened?   Marketing may succumb to reality.

Several years ago in a National Neurosurgical meeting, a presenter, who was a reputable neurosurgeon, discussed a spinal technique with a 70% success rate. Apparently, this is how the majority of such surgeries are performed in China, allegedly for economic reasons. And he started using it here, discussed its roll In managing disk herniations.

I commented to the audience that this technique was used by myself thirty years ago, but I stopped developing it, because it "only" had a success rate of 70% (compared to another technique with 90-95% success).

He answered, that for such a procedure, this rate was quite acceptable.

How can you argue that?

Fashion lives !

But I already said too much.

I suppose like much of my brethren, I'm very judgmental…comes with the territory. There's an old neurosurgical saying, "I may not always be right, but I'm always certain." Gotta be that way.

I may leave the reader perhaps, a little perplexed.
Life is that way sometimes. Much as I admire my profession and my colleagues, one can always see room for improvement, some overdue.

The parting words for any budding neurosurgeon are: Perfection "and" Respect. Oh, and you better remain committed to a life of learning (thank god for that opportunity) and physical demands.

Best wishes,

POSTSCRIPT

Interesting voyage, no?

I trust the narrative hasn't been too challenging. I certainly understand how my personal "revelations" might be upsetting for some. I don't wish to imply this was a traditional path for any individual in medicine. Truth is, there are many, some I am sure, even more novel than mine. What I hoped to impart is the "sensation" physically and emotionally, of my journey and how many, many patient lives have effected me, even my family. The trip was awesome.

But in this regard, I "volunteered" to have the life I chose. And while I would do it again, my son didn't volunteer to having the phone constantly ringing throughout the night, as an infant, a child and teenager. Or, a father sometimes absent, despite best efforts.

And my wife who saw me through, and without her assistance, I would have truly failed Did she comprehend the magnitude of our decision, in the beginning? For their contributions, I am extremely grateful.

Finally my patients, did they know how committed I was to their welfare?

Did they understand when I had to prioritize a more critically ill patient, or ran behind in my office, because no patients showed up the first hour, then they all arrived together. Or, if their results did not meet expectations, that all possibilities were considered, with risks rewards-ratio calculated throughout their evaluation and treatment?

Did the families recognize my commitment to their loved ones? I can only Hope so.

I took pride in my belief that I was the best in what I did.
I suspect most neurosurgeons feel the same way.
They like me, have to continually challenge themselves.
Could we have done that better?

It is one that we embrace, but sometimes even as physicians, can minimize the importance of our decisions, which alter lives.

If I could be granted a professional wish, it would be that patients and their families would know how much their lives really meant to me and mine.
They made the Journey well worth it.

www.ingramcontent.com/pod-product-compliance
Lightning Source LLC
Chambersburg PA
CBHW080544220526
45466CB00010B/3025